CREATE THE AMAZING DENTAL EXPERIENCE

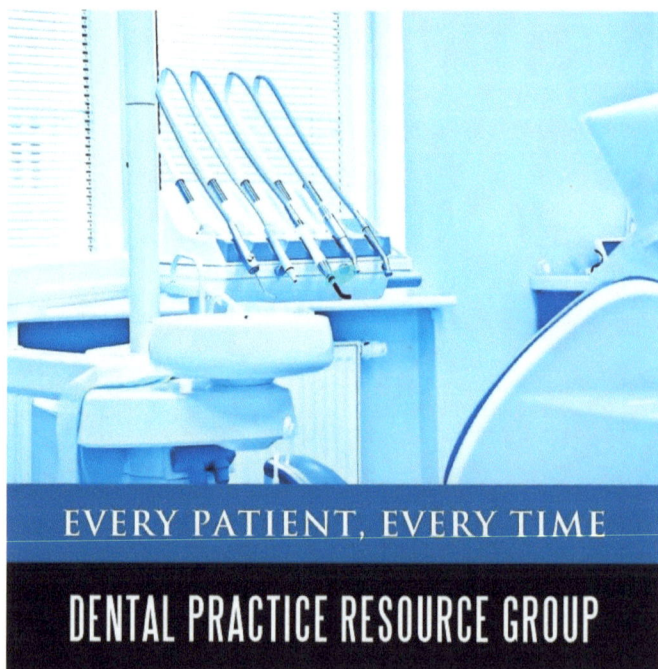

EVERY PATIENT, EVERY TIME

DENTAL PRACTICE RESOURCE GROUP

Creating An Amazing Dental Experience

Every Patient, Every Time

Dental Practice Resource Group
Mitchel Schwindt

Beginning To Amaze

Introduction

You have the education and training to provide high quality dental care. Everyday, your team strives to deliver the promise of an amazing experience to every patient. While this is a laudable goal, having a tool chest full of strategies, tactics and techniques makes the goal a reality.

Reading this book will reward those that implement even just a few of the ideas contained. Highlight and mark it all up with thoughts and iterations on how these tactics will work in your practice environment. Plan team meetings around specific ideas and capitalize on delivering an experience that sets your practice apart from the rest.

Continually Invest In The Culture Of The Practice

Defining the precise culture of your practice in words is difficult but essential. You must get this first step right.

Without some planning, strategizing and direction, the culture will become amorphous, wrong or disappear altogether.

Be intentional - create, iterate and invest wholeheartedly in the culture of your practice.

Careful crafting of culture will hold your team and practice together solidifying your office as the ideal team of which to belong.

Although the word is used a lot these days, it's worth defining what we mean by 'culture.' Your corporate culture is the tone that your organization takes, formal, relaxed, or informal. It's also how the management (you) deals with staff. Do you see yourself in a formal relationship, in family, etc? All of these things will inform your culture.

The result is a powerful energy and undercurrent to ensure each patient has an amazing experience - every time.

Clarify The Mission

Intention, focus, and clarity must all be utilized. The most important part of establishing a culture relies on having a precise definition of the practice's mission.

Define your culture around how best to provide an amazing experience for each patient at each visit.

Be Prepared to Experiment Every Day

Resist the temptation to 'set it and forget it'. Adapt a flexible mindset and understand that change is constant. Not every day or every patient is identical.

Constant experimentation and creativity will ensure your practice continues to deliver the type of experience you want every patient to have.

Empower your team to take matters into their hands to exceed patient expectations. Promoting this mindset and culture openly fosters a sense of belonging and achievement among each team member.

Understand that not every idea will work, but being a bit scientific about it and tracking results will create a new paradigm in patient experience setting your practice apart from the rest.

Assign a 'scientist' from your team to report on the results of these experiments. The what, why and how of consistently delivering an incredible patient experience will become crystal clear and unique to your practice and team.

What They See

Follow The Leader

Although the memories of playing this game are at the far reaches of my memory, it still has some valuable lessons. Let me share a quick story about this point.

Six years ago, I was working at a corporate type office and noted a pervasive sour mood. We received little administrative support and the team felt overworked, underpaid and underappreciated. It wasn't always that way, but a slow current of negativity seeped in and was threatening to destroy morale for good. I had even noticed a shift in my normally upbeat demeanor. After complaining to my wife and friends about it for several months, the truth finally hit me square in the face. The problem was me.

As leader of this group totaling 5 clinicians and thirty staff, my own bias and negativity had unknowingly spread to all the corners of the practice. What I realized during some long nights of thinking was that I had to change, and fast. I made a resolve to put on my game face each and every day and to keep the negative thoughts and snide comments to myself. In short, I just sucked it up. Almost immediately, I noticed a change in some of the key players. The mood was lighter and our team seemed better able to cope with or shrug off the daily problems that are unavoidable in a busy practice such as ours.

Behind the scenes, I began to work arduously with administration to get the support and appreciation we deserved. Like most bureaucratic things, change was slow. Over the next two years, our situation improved appreciably. I learned a lot during those stressful few years and realized that eight years in the corporate mill cranking through patients as fast as humanly possible was no longer tenable. I tendered my resignation with mixed emotion since leaving behind friends is always hard, but it was the right decision. That was six years ago, and I'm happy to say that I don't regret that decision one bit.

Do This

- Identify who are the leaders in your practice - lead hygienist, office manager, social media?
- Empower team members to "own" the practice
- Determine activities and educational opportunities to build leaders and leadership
-

Own The Place

Empowering each team member to feel like someone important will create an amazing culture in any clinic or organization. Giving autonomy over small decisions frees up your plate to focus on what you do best - dentistry. Depending on the size of your staff and comfort level, consider the next few examples and see what you can come up with in your practice.

Our office manager has the Ben Franklin stamp and can make any decision for the good of the practice up to $100 without checking or clearing it with any of the dentist partners. We let the receptionist have a similar, but scaled down freedom of up to $20. Often, they don't spend even that, but a latte or a carwash card can go a long way to soother the ruffled feather of an annoyed patient.

Do You Trust?

Judgment is a crucial piece of growth. Mistakes can and will happen. How you respond will make all the difference.

Take a moment and think about parenting. Our goal is to guide without controlling and protect without stifling growth. Shifting the balance too far in either direction will result in rebellion or danger.

Adopt a similar approach when dealing with your team. Mistakes are always a vital part of the learning process. Try shifting your view from the idea that mistakes are the sign of a weak team member to capitalizing on the event as a learning process. Thomas Edison is quoted as saying "I haven't failed. I've just found 10,000 ways that don't work".

Instilling confidence in your team drives them to make more good decisions than bad. Not all mistakes are preventable, so resist the temptation to look through the "retrospectoscope."

Do This

- Encourage decision making and accept that not all will be perfect
- Let your team know you value and trust them
- Use mistakes as a learning opportunity
- Let the trust your team feels from you will translate into a more cohesive practice
-

Post Mortem

As chapter one pointed out, mistakes are inevitable. Consider creating a system for dissecting the mistakes and teasing out learning points. Having a clear understanding of what happened goes a long way to preventing the same mistake in the future. It is often a series of missteps along the way that resulted in a faulty decision.

Next, use the same system to analyze the big wins.

Savor the positive experiences and patient encounters. Congratulate the team on positive reviews and social media shares and shout-outs. After the cheers die down, conduct an instant replay. See if your team can recall the specifics of what created a magical experience for the patient. Was it a simple act of kindness? Taking a moment to listen to a problem or concern with extra attention? Maybe someone in the office complimented the patient or recalled an important event in the patient's life. By teasing out the specifics, it becomes easier to reproduce an amazing experience for every patient.

Happy patients talk about your practice, and word of mouth is a powerful referral tool.

Do This
- Apply the same system to dissect moments of excellence
- Celebrate the wins, but learn from them as well
- Rinse and repeat - create evangelists for your practice

Embracing The Curve

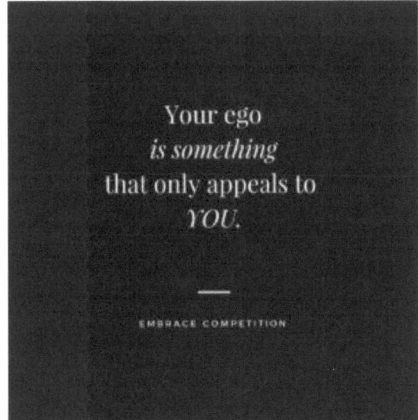

The ego often gets in the way of life. Jealousy is a formidable foe.

Business is a lot like life and separating the two is nearly impossible as we have so much invested in our practices.

While the temptation to criticize often surfaces out of jealousy, learn to make friends with your competition. By adopting an abundance mindset, you are inviting the universe to conspire to grow your practice.

Without diving into the deep end of philosophy, consider befriending your competitors. Learn from their successes as well as mistakes.

The next time you see an ad for a competing dental office put aside the judgment and comparison. Take an honest look at what they did well. How would the ad make you feel if you were a potential patient? Solicit impressions from your staff, friends and family.

Next, apply this information when creating your own ads or marketing materials. As we've said before, the wheel doesn't have to be reinvented every time. It is perfectly acceptable to let others do the heavy lifting at times.

The next time you attend a meeting or continuing education event, invite someone from a practice you admire to coffee or lunch. Be open, honest and exchange information. There is value in seeing how others think and approach managing their practice.

Do This
- Learn about your competition and capitalize on what you do best
- Adopt an abundance mindset. It's not a zero-sum game.
- By exchanging information, you can capitalize on your competition's limitations and exploit your own strengths
- Embrace the learning curve and keep an open mind about new or different ideas
-

Don't Act Your Age

I am reasonably confident that how you practice dentistry is similar to how you trained during dental school.

I am not, however, as convinced that every practice has embraced the changing times and power of the internet and all its nuances.

The topic at hand is the internet and social media. Long past are the days where having a sign on the front of your office is enough. Everyone and everything is on the web and discoverability is a driving factor in your success.

Embrace Those Who Love The Future

The chances are that you prefer reading and taking courses on the latest restorative technique or materials or are branching out into implant dentistry or another niche. There is simply not enough time to be an expert at everything - including the web.

Hiring a staff member with experience and skill in social media can be a boon for your dental practice. We have several assistants who love Pinterest, Twitter, and Instagram. Why sweat over how to use these current platforms when you may already have someone on your team who likes this sort of thing. Allocate time and add a financial piece to it if appropriate and turn them loose.

Set up some ground rules about what types of things you would like to see. Focus a staff meeting on a strategy to engage and celebrate current patients while attracting new patients. Run contests. Reward the cavity-free kids club. Host a local event, like a 5K race and share anything your team participates in while supporting the local community. The options are endless.

Our practice is continually pitched by "experts" charging thousands to do what our staff already loves to do. By adding a fun task to their job description, we have been able to retain and reward some of the most enthusiastic team members to date. Do some research before hiring an outside firm. Look at what type of content they generate and see if your staff are up to the task. No one knows your office better than your staff and patients.

Do This:
- Survey your patients and staff to find out where they hang out online
- Pick one or two social media platforms and start engaging and sharing
- Choose a staff member to help manage these accounts
- Share, educate and entertain your followers

Self Examination

Have You Checked In On Your Practice Lately?

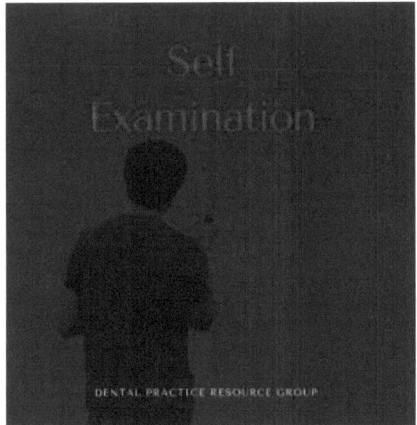

In the last chapter, we talked about sharing and creating an encouraging message to both rewards existing clients and entices new patients. But how do you know if it's working?

Monitor Yourself

This is easier than it sounds. With the advent of Facebook statistics, it's simple to see how often people like your content or shared it, but what about the rest of the web?

There is a wealth of programs and services available to monitor your efforts and brand. We use Google Alerts, Mention, Buffer, and Tweetdeck. Some are free, others offer upgraded accounts. I'll share a list of other options in a moment.

The bottom line is that you need to monitor your brand. Engage with a thank you and pay attention to the criticism. A word of caution: ignore the trolls. There are always those who get off on posting hateful words to cause others angst. Use your intuition to discern what are real issues and complaints and make it an opportunity to learn.

A few other strategies to help your practice reputation:

- Contact site owners if the post violates the site's policies. This may get it removed.
- Create positive and valuable content and the less favorable tend to sift to the bottom over time.
- Understand that you will not 'correct' a naysayer's opinion or feelings online. Avoid getting into a shouting match.
- Realize that most of the negative comments come from a minority but, unfortunately, a vocal minority.
- If they are, in fact, patients of record, engage in the normal social channels and keep the conversation offline. You   remember a little thing called HIPPA?
-

Social Media Monitoring Tools

- Tweetdeck
- Twitter search
- Hootsuite
- Mention
- Talkwalker
- Google Alerts

- Buffer
- Facebook..of course

What tools do you currently use? Don't stress about picking the perfect tool as technology changes. The point is to start if you haven't already. You need to know what others are saying about you and your dental practice.

The Power of One

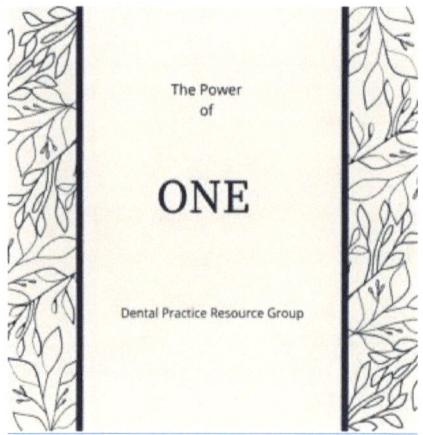

In today's modern world of excess, it is very easy to become obsessed with more. Looking at quantity instead of quality is a temptation many cannot resist. The value of one patient must not be overlooked.

Consider for a moment, what brings joy to your day? What type of patient interactions are rewarding and leave your team with a sense of satisfaction, purpose, and happiness? Just as any successful coach wants "A" players on the team and not "C stringers," the same concept applies to your dental practice.

By delivering an amazing dental experience, your patients become loyal brand advocates and repeat customers and are more likely to accept your treatment plan. You want to keep these patients and encourage their friends and family to become patients, as well.

What emotion do you experience when a patient accepts your treatment plan of 3 crowns and wants to get started right away? How about the patient that fights every decision you make and argues about the cost of everything? Or the patient that refuses to floss and never keeps their cleaning appointments, but then harasses you on weekends for their emergency toothaches? Which do you prefer as your primary patient base?

The answer is clear, and the value of your "A" patients goes beyond the financial aspect.

Patients are your customers, and each has a lifetime value to your practice. Keeping existing valuable patients is much easier than recruiting new patients and starting from scratch.

Going back to previous chapters, the ability for your team to solve issues on the fly and keep patients happy is crucial. Solving patient problems has a positive emotional impact on all involved and helps the patient maintain a positive impression of your entire practice. Reinforcing positive experiences fosters loyalty. Going "above and beyond" and exceeding expectations will set your practice apart from the competition.

Do This

- Make sure your team understands the lifetime value of patients
- Empower your team to make decisions to keep these patients happy
- Role play and create a playbook or script for managing difficult patient scenarios
-

Knowing on Purpose

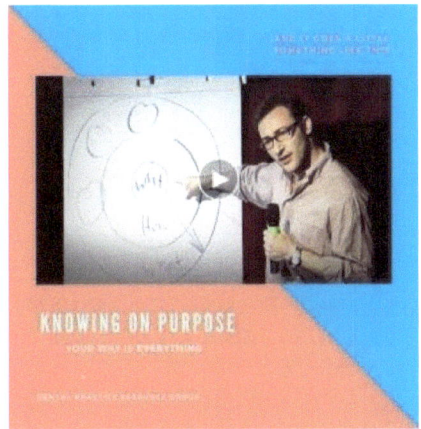

I am sure you consider your practice a success on several levels, but have you clearly defined what makes you a success?

Once you clearly define your **why**, the chances of reaching higher and consistent levels of success are exponentially improved. By knowing your 'why,' your team can deliver a consistently amazing dental experience for all your patients.

If you haven't heard of Simon Sinek, I encourage you to watch his TED talk here:

http://dentalpracticeresourcegroup.com/yourwhy

Our office has defined the factors most important for our success. They also align with our **why**.

- Patient experience
- Product
- Place
- Promotion
- Plan

Patients are the keystone of every dental practice and by ensuring that every patient has a positive and rewarding experience, our number one goal is met. Caring for patients is why you chose dentistry, after all.

The products our office produces are more than fillings, crowns, and implants. Consider the patient as a product as well. Through education, positive reinforcement, and patience, your team is literally creating a healthier human being.

Think back to the last time you tried a new restaurant or checked into a different hotel. I'll bet you remember those places that stood out above the rest. Often, this is because of how you felt. Take care and craft an office environment that speaks to the patient on a different level. Instead of a sterile aesthetic and uncomfortable chairs spend some time and currency creating an environment where patients feel at home. Several patients stop by at regular intervals for a cup of coffee or to share a personal story with the front office staff. This occurs when they aren't scheduled for an appointment and is a testament to the environment and culture we have created.

Promotion goes beyond marketing efforts to get your name out into the community. Creating contests and opportunities to promote the success of your patients are great ways to promote loyalty to your practice. A few ideas we have implemented:

- Cavity free kids - 100$ saving bond & movie tickets

- Guess the number of teeth. We fill a jar with candy teeth around Halloween and patients guess to win prizes.

- Community races are a great way to promote health, build camaraderie and share your practice with the community. We have a race team made up of patients sporting fun free t-shirts with our practice name and logo. Each racer gets a goodie bag with healthy treats, toothbrush, floss and fun stuff donated by other community businesses.

Planning is essential. Don't expect one person to do it all and coordinate every idea and event. Enlist team support and buy-in to create a cohesive practice environment. Just like long-term treatment planning is vital to your success, getting your team to brainstorm and create fun and innovative ways to reward your patients is a powerful way to grow your practice.

Intentionally Bad

Don't Be A Jack Of All

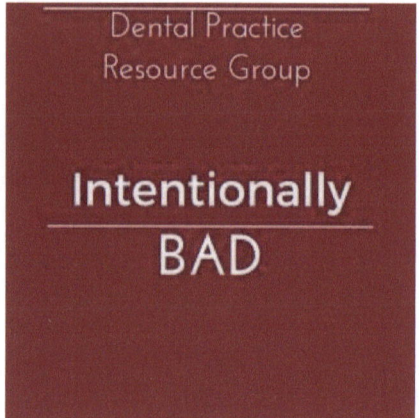

Today's thinking is tearing apart the fabric of the Western World. We force our children to attempt to master every subject. Self-help experts encourage working on weaknesses. This approach leads to mediocrity across all aspects of life.

Our emphasis needs to be on creating an amazing experience for every patient every time. While the general practice of dentistry allows competence in many procedures and techniques, no single dentist can be excellent at everything. Nor should they be. I have talked to many colleagues who ruminate over cases that didn't go particularly well. This is normal but consider the phrase, jack of all trades - master of none.

Do you want that phrase to define your practice?

By focusing on your talents and intentionally being bad at your weaknesses is an opportunity to set yourself apart. Once you get over the emotional baggage of referring cases that don't serve your patient or yourself well, you are free to pursue excellence in the area most exciting and rewarding to you professionally.

Your patients will thank you once they understand the rationale. Several of my closest friends loathe molar endo and refer all cases out of their practices. Patients are met with an amazing experience, and a skilled endodontist can complete the case in a fraction of the time. They return to your practice for what you do best.

Not every potential patient should be your patient. Your growing reputation will self-select some patients, and others will gravitate to your practice for various reasons. Be prepared to say no to some and to fire other patients. Life is too short to deal with the emotional drain produced by toxic patients. Make the strategic decision to deliver fantastic dental care, but also to be happy and fulfilled.

Continue to differentiate your practice based on what you are already good at. Fire bad patients and acknowledge that you will be bad at some procedures or techniques. After that is out of the way, you are free to capitalize on your unique talents and skills.

Do This

- • Choose to be intentionally bad (at some things)
- • Accept that perfection doing everything is not attainable
- • Fire bad patients
- • Take inventory of what you are already good at and become great at those things

Fire Everyone

Be As You Are

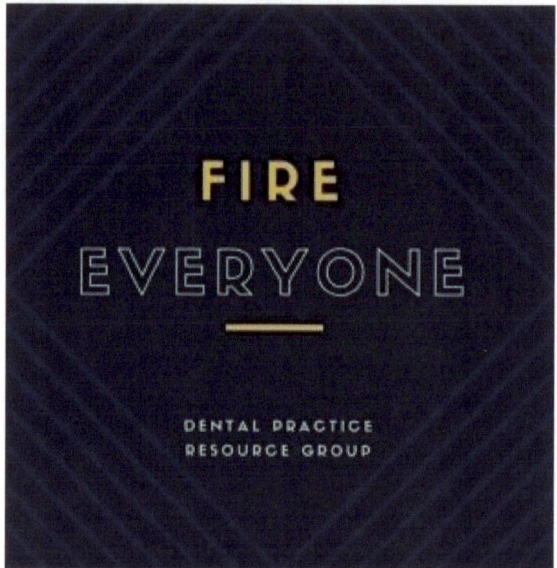

Do you want to throw touchdown passes or kick field goals? If you think you can do both, then you are stuck back in the glory days of high school.

It's time to step up to the pros.

Being an effective leader of any team requires developing a strategy for the personal growth of each member of the office staff. While staff positions have clearly defined roles and responsibilities, individuals have unique aspirations and interests. Make it a priority to discover the unique talents that lay hidden among your staff.

Fire Yourself!

If you don't like posting to social media, fire yourself. Most likely, a member of your team loves Facebook and Pinterest or Instagram and would be more than happy to take over this task. Consider the pros and cons of having the office manager blindly assign tasks vs. asking team members to step up to what interests them. I'm constantly surprised when the most outgoing staff member has a passion for microbiology and all things OSHA. Who knew? She was tickled pink to take on this role for the practice.

Allowing our team to express their areas of interest and declare strengths fosters job satisfaction and a sense of belonging. We encourage our staff to share their ideas and, when necessary, sit down and pull it out of them. It makes sense on a visceral level to help a staff member become great at an area of interest, rather than focusing only on improving deficiencies.

Do This

- Develop a plan for promoting personal and professional growth for each member of the team
- Focus on your strengths and fire yourself from tasks when necessary
- Ask - don't assume that you understand the specific interests of individuals
- Fire team members from tasks performed in a mediocre fashion and reassign to areas of strength and interest

Culture Club

Crafting Culture

Your Culture Club

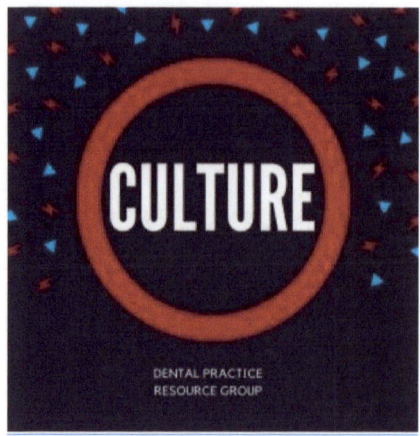

"Culture is the arts elevated to a set of beliefs." - Thomas Wolfe

Look into the most successful companies and you'll find an amazing culture. Focus on your employees and witness a sustainable culture that celebrates patients and team members. Treat your staff as you want to be treated, not as cogs in the dental machine.

As the leader, you are primarily responsible for setting the tone in the practice and articulating a clear vision of the culture. Whatever you create inside the team will be felt outside, by the patients and community.

Think back to an experience where you were amazed by the energy or vibe of a business. Maybe it was a restaurant or an event. What was the single element that stood out? More than likely, it was how the place made you feel. The culture created an infectious energy that was impossible to miss.

By carefully crafting your culture, a system is formed that inspires and motivates everyone on the team. Maintaining an active and positive culture is crucial for retaining talented staff.

Do This:
- Carefully craft the unique culture that personifies your values and beliefs
- Create a positive culture that rewards and retains great talent
- Be the leader and set an example of what the culture looks, feels and tastes like
-

Cheers

Everybody Knows Your Name

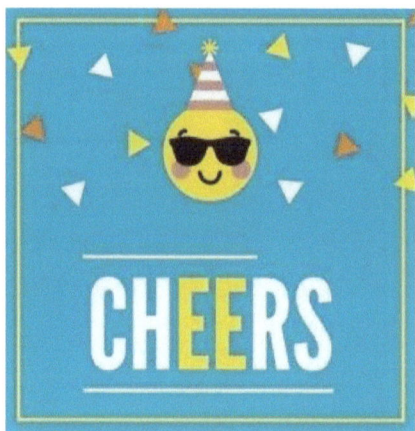

Although I may be dating myself a bit, the reference to Cheers it too powerful to resist.

The characters of the famous Boston bar Cheers share their lives with each other while drinking or working at the bar.

Consider this phrase from the theme song of Cheers:

Sometimes you want to go to a place where everybody knows your name, and they are always glad you came.

https://www.youtube.com/watch?v=h-mi0r0LpXo

We spend so much of our lives at work, why not develop a culture that puts the team at the center and creates a positive setting where everybody loves to come to work?

A top-down approach where you set the example of how to treat everyone on the team will spill over into how the team treats each patient. Implement the "Golden Rule" in your dental office just as you would in everyday life.

Next, focus on the driving theme of your practice. What single statement defines how you want the practice to be known for?

-Gentle

-Modern

-Helpful

-Compassionate

-Progressive

Our practice focuses on providing gentle care. It has become an internal slogan for our team. We treat each other with kindness and understanding for each person's uniqueness and gifts. The same acceptance is extended to our patients. Through constant reinforcement, this attitude has permeated every corner of the office and consistently creates a sense of calm for our patients.

Every team member is aligned with this purpose, and it is fused into the DNA of our practice. Team members are treated very well, and an attitude of mutual respect has created the best place to work, practice dentistry, and deliver gentle, yet amazing, patient care.

Do This:

- • Live the "Golden Rule" – Do unto others as you would have done to you.
- • Set an active example of the core principle driving the practice
- • Create the best place to work for your team - They cannot amaze patients if they are miserable
-

Own This

Why You Need To Own This?

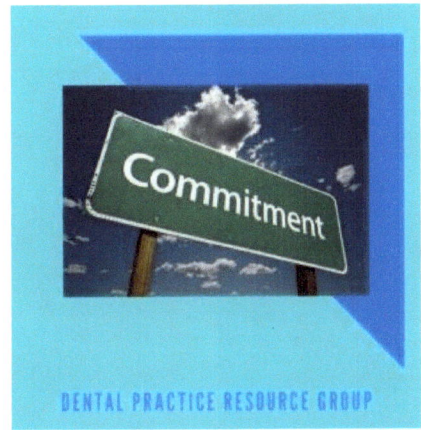

Empowering patients to be their own best oral health advocates is a noble mission everyone on the team must own.

Educating patients, parents, and families is the cornerstone of building a solid understanding of the oral-systemic health link. Don't expect patients to get it right off the bat. Some of your team may not understand the full impact of this approach for maximizing health and longevity.

Be creative and let your team members use their own brand of education. The message is best delivered in a manner consistent with their personal communication abilities and style. Forcing fancy words or adherence to a script often results in push-back and lack-luster learning for your patients. Encourage each team member to create a unique message that resonates with their values and incorporates the essential message of how oral health impacts all aspects of health.

Do This:

- Devote several education sessions to bring the team up to speed on the current trends in oral-systemic health

- Rephrase and remove modifiers such as a "small" or "minor" issue, i.e., gum disease has a whole body impact and is tied   to heart disease, diabetes and brain health. None of these is small or minor.

- Plan a staff trip to a conference or invite local experts for a "lunch and learn" session.

10X

Success vs. Failure

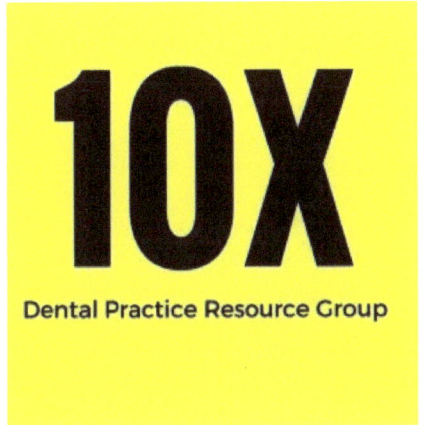

Effort is often the only difference between success and failure. One of my favorite books is 10X by Grant Cardone. While you may not all like his speaking style, his message resonates the truth about what separates out the most successful from the rest.

It is that extra effort, the extra mile, which separates champions from those who just show up. The same concept applies to every day in a dental practice.

Patients make requests and many times the off-the-cuff responses are, "I don't know," or "I'll have to get back to you." This is a simple strategy to ignore or decline a request, without seeing if it is possible or feasible.

Team members who put forth the effort to solve patients' problems build an unstoppable force of loyalty and evangelism for your practice. Give your team the authority to creatively solve patient requests and let them take ownership and pride in being problem-solvers, instead of excuse makers.

.

Do This

- Solve problems instead of offer excuses
- Empower the team to be creative to find solutions
- Accept the cost of solving problems as an economic weapon in providing loyalty and creating "practice evangelists"
-

One For All

The Face Of Your Practice

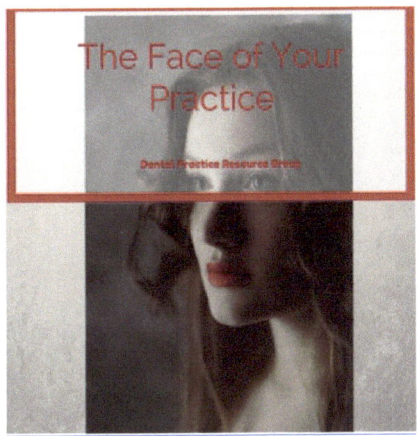

"Please be seated with your seatbelt fastened." These were the last words I heard before drifting off to a fitful sleep aboard an airline I don't usually fly.

Battling a cold, I had to finish the final leg of a consulting trip and was grateful to get a seat on the oversold flight. Like many, I am a creature of habit and fly Delta whenever I can. This day was different in many ways.

Feeling a jolt of pain sear through my neck and shoulder, I awoke to the flight attendant jerking on my seatback. "Sir, your seat needs to be all the way upright before landing."

Wow. What a rude awakening! I had developed a kink in my neck after falling asleep in an awkward position in a broken seat. It wouldn't recline or return to full upright, no matter what I did to it. If she had only taken a few moments to rouse me and ask, the outcome of my opinion would have been much different. Instead, I labeled this airline in a permanently negative fashion. All from the actions of one staff member.

The point to drive home is this: that patients do business with your practice, but, in reality, it all boils down to one-on-one interactions. When a team member delivers an amazing experience, the patient labels your entire practice as amazing. At any given moment, a single team member is the sole representative of you and your practice. Fair or not, it's reality.

Perform periodic assessments of how well each team member represents your brand. Opportunities for improvement will undoubtedly surface, and this is the perfect chance to strengthen weak links. With some work and coaching, even the weakest team member can consistently deliver an amazing experience to the patient.

Do This:
- Use a secret shopper type service to assess your team's performance
- Devote time to role-playing or sharing scenarios during team meetings
- Deconstruct both good and bad patient encounters and learn from both
- Ensure that even the weakest team member has the tools to deliver an amazing patient experience

image credit:
roksolana-zasiadko

Playbook Edit

On The Fly

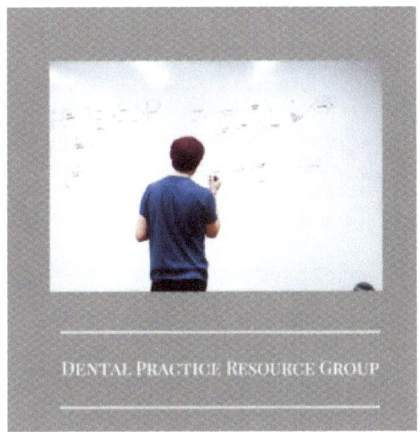

Anyone familiar with the game of football knows about the coveted "playbook." This strategy book lays out the ground rules of how to conduct specific plays for specific situations to get specific results. We have a similar playbook our team uses as the framework for conducting business.

You know, as well as I, that patients and illness don't read, nor care, about the playbook. That's what makes practicing so stimulating.

Edit On The Fly

Most of our team is cross-trained in several operational aspects of running a busy dental office. To lay the groundwork, copays are due before treatment is rendered. It's spelled out clearly in our policy manual.

Due to an illness, one of our newest team members found herself at the front desk and demanding a copayment before service from a patient. The patient forgot her purse and admitted that it was a simple oversight on her part, but demanded to be seen as her work schedule is very tight. This was the only appointment she could get away to as a busy midlevel executive. Our team member insisted that without payment, she would not be seen that day. Fortunately, another team member overheard and offered some guidance.

The patient happened to be one of our most loyal customers and had been coming to the practice for nearly ten years. Our culture puts the patient first and allows the team to use their best judgment to deliver amazing patient experiences. We also encourage coaching and mentoring by senior staff to ensure a consistent experience across all aspects of patient flow through the practice.

Do This:
- Encourage use of best judgment to solve patient issues
- Adopt a mentoring mindset where senior staff can guide junior staff in creating amazing patient experiences
- Having a patient first (customer first) mindset lets patients know you are their advocate
-

What Word

Word?

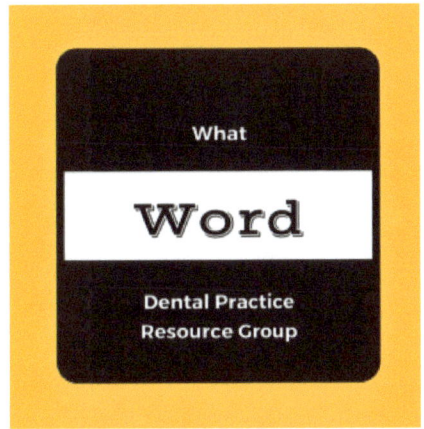

A single word wields power. Replace any word or modify the blank in the following sentence and everything changes.

I _____ you.

Shifting focus and adjusting the way we talk to one another has the power to transform the culture of your office. Replacing the label of "employee" with "team member" has made a tremendous difference in our practice. New hires often note a feeling of teamwork and an atmosphere more welcoming than they'd experienced in past office settings.

Although decision-making and treatment planning are complex, the patient is the boss and drives all final decisions. Acknowledging this fact, and shifting both mindset and communication around this concept, moves the culture of a practice and refocuses it on a patient-first approach. I'm not advocating calling a patient "the boss," but thinking of them as part of your team triggers the mental shift necessary for a long-term partnership of success.

Changing how words are used causes attitude to follow. This will be evident to your patients, and we often receive comments such as:

"I love this office."

"They make me feel like my opinion matters."

"All of the staff are gracious and respect my choices."

Do This

- Analyze how your team refers to patients
- Use or create an alternative with positive implications - friends, team, family, etc.
- Changing words can shift the entire culture of the practice
- Develop a sense of teamwork and scrap the boss-employee terminology

Two Jobs

The Power Of Two

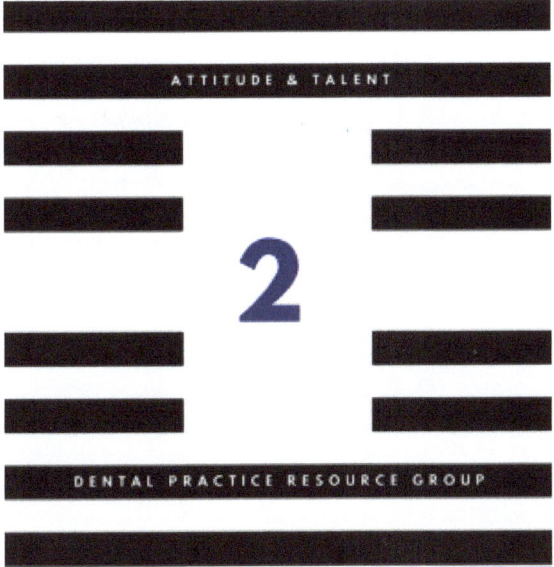

Whether you like it or not, every aspect and every team member is under constant scrutiny. Your patient/customers are guests in your practice and must be treated as such.

When your practice adopts a patient-first mindset as the primary driver of behavior, patients will take notice. Then they will share their perceptions on Facebook, Yelp, Google, and wherever else they feel like sharing.

More than One

When the practice culture embraces a patient-first mindset, every team member automatically takes on another job as the patient-first advocate. In the business world, this is referred to as customer service.

When current and new hires understand the importance of keeping patients happy, this task often becomes self-evident. Every point of patient contact in the practice is an opportunity for ensuring excellent patient-first service. Empower your team to do the job they were hired to do, but also to take care of patient comfort and manage impressions and expectations.

Simple examples:

- The hygienist takes the last cup of coffee. Instead of waiting for other staff to notice, she immediately brews a fresh pot so that patients in the waiting room don't have to wait for coffee.

- The assistant notices some trash on the sidewalk on the way into the office. She understands that patients will see it and, even though it's external to the practice, it can negatively impact the impression of the office. She picks it up without a second thought and grabs a stray napkin on her way through the waiting room. All this occurs before she officially starts her workday.

- The front desk receptionist is busy taking calls and checking in patients, but notices the significant other of a patient seems uncomfortable. She steps away from the desk to offer assistance. It turns out that he twisted his ankle walking up the steps in a rush to get his physically-challenged wife to this appointment. She offers an ice pack and helps him prop his sprained ankle up on a chair while he waits.

These seemingly minor acts are outside the scope of formal job descriptions but have an impact on the practice's reputation. A team who willingly accepts two jobs ensures that every patient experiences a caring and comfortable environment.

Do This:

Encourage all team members to visualize patients as friends and family

Promote the concept of two jobs and ensure that patients always come first

Understand that even if not directly interacting with a patient, each team member is supporting the patient-first culture and helping other team members accomplish that goal

Different Flavors

Embrace The Difference

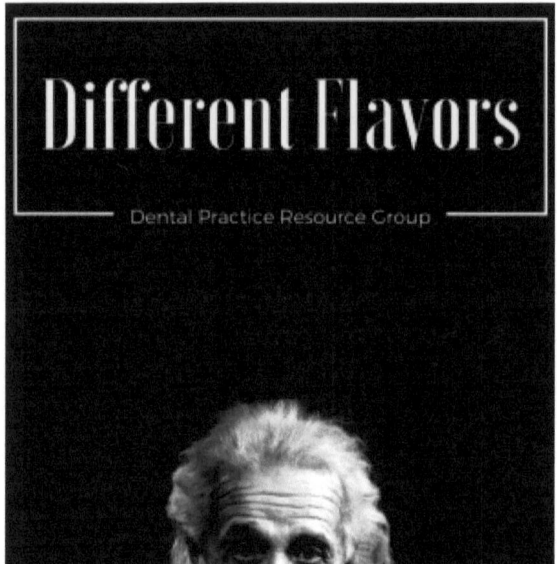

The power of a team lies in its members. Not just sheer numbers but in uniqueness. Just as one size or shade does not fit all anterior composites, the same applies to a successful team.

While everyone needs to endorse the underlying culture, the means to accomplish this are nearly limitless. That is the beauty of having a diverse team comprised of uniqueness.

Encouraging team members to solve problems based on their personal experience and strengths reinforces a sense of accomplishment and belonging. It also allows your practice to win by solving problems utilizing divergent thinking.

"We cannot solve our problems with the same level of thinking that created them."
-Albert Einstein

Celebrate the successes of the team and practice by embracing the different personalities, skills, talents, and opinions of each member.

Do This:

- Reinforce the core culture statement, but let team members utilize their uniqueness to fulfill that mission
- Consider the power of originality when building your team
- Relive past successes when a divergent way of thinking solved a patient issue
-

Favorite Cookie

What Do You Love About Your Favorite Cookie?

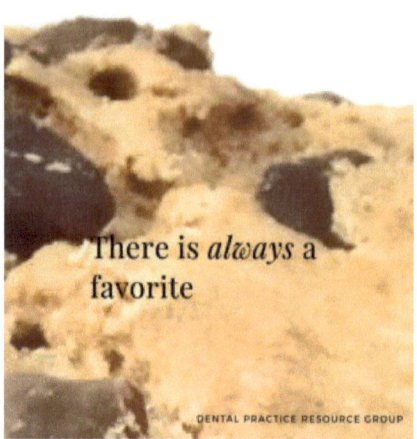

The chances are that you have a single favorite flavor of something. Maybe it's a cookie, burger, or wine, but one thing is for certain: You expect a certain consistency. In fact, you demand it. If your brand fails on this account, you will pick a different one.

The same principle applies to your practice. Patients learn to know, like, and trust you. They have tasted the cookie and liked everything about it. Change the recipe and chances are you will be met with some unhappy faces.

What usually happens is what should **usually** happen.

Most people, patients included, dislike change. Unless there is a compelling reason, consider the consequences of any changes.

When change is necessary, take the time to explain and forewarn them. Patients appreciate being kept in the loop. Often, the honest reason for change more than makes up for any inconvenience or concern.

Years ago, I contemplated a career as a pilot. I can still recall my instructor harping on me to follow the checklist and not go off of memory. Commercial pilots perform everything by checklists with the result of system-wide safety, efficiency, and consistency. The same process can be utilized in the dental practice.

Sit down with your team and follow a new patient as they flow into the practice. The steps are largely the same for the majority of new patients. Document what happens or what you want to happen when they open your office door for the first time. Walk through an entire visit and follow them out the door. What happens next? Does your office have a follow-up protocol in place?

By understanding the processes at play in your practice, your team can develop a consistency that patients will appreciate and find comfort. Taking the time to map it all out guides your team to play the same game and also makes transitioning new team members consistent and much easier.

Do This

- Create systems and ensure the team knows and follows the protocol
- Document the process with a chart or mindmap
- Accept when protocols and procedures break down or no longer function
- Periodically assess areas for process improvement, and then educate and inform all involved, including the patients

Options for Documenting Processes

http://mindnode.com/

https://www.lucidchart.com/

Brain Dump

Unload Your Mind

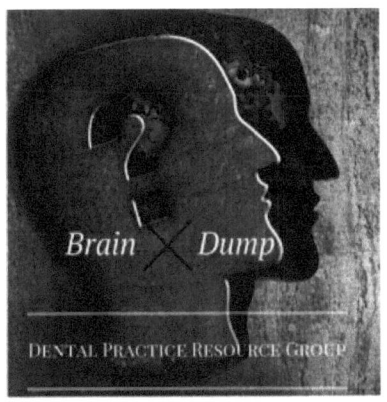

Great ideas are lurking in the minds of your team. Your job as the leader is to tease these ideas out. Create a culture that rewards sharing ideas and prohibits negativity.

Have you ever observed a second-grade classroom? Notice what happens when the teacher asks a question? All hands go up. Somewhere along our development that all shifts. Now, we are reluctant to offer opinion or insights. Is it possible to regain that fearlessness?

Rewarding Thoughts

Through encouragement, and with the strict adoption of a no-criticism policy, it is possible, even likely, that your team will share what's on their minds.

Consider starting with small requests for ideas during team meetings. Gauge the level of response and praise those who speak up. Unfortunately, I've had the experience on several occasions to be met with blank stares. Suddenly, everyone is interested in the pattern on the carpet.

One possible solution is to solicit ideas ahead of the meeting by requesting each department write down three ideas about how to improve the practice or solve a particular problem. Invite free thinking and creativity.

Another option is to utilize a simple whiteboard. In one of our practices, the team uses a whiteboard in the lunch and team meeting area. Anyone can write an idea or suggestion on the board. Then it's discussed at the next team meeting. Sometimes, the idea is so good that it's pulled into the morning huddle and implemented that same day.

Do This

- Create an incentive or reward for idea sharing
- Cultivate a no-criticism mindset provide alternatives for sharing ideas - an idea board, dream board, team suggestion box, etc.

Need some help? Try this guide for your Dental Practice. https://gum.co/smile5

photo credit: bigstock-Human-brain-open-with-question-52652104

Story Time

What Story Do You Want Your Patients To Tell?

"**Time is a good story teller**" - Irish Proverb

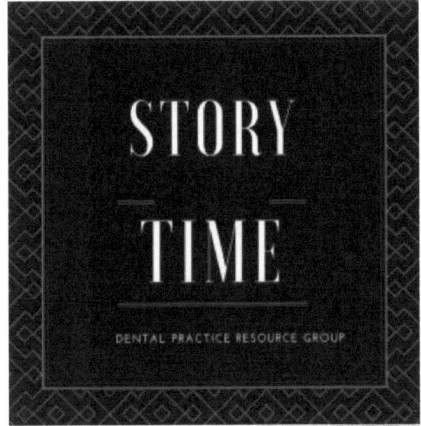

The stories your patients tell creates a distinct flavor to your culture. By giving them the script, you are well on your way to a narrative that cultivates pride and drives more patients to your door.

I have a close friend who happens to be an amazing cook and host. His dinner parties are an incredible event, and an invitation is to be treasured. No doubt he has culinary chops, but it goes well beyond that.

When I asked him how he creates such amazing events, his response surprised me.

He related that it's like writing a good story. One has to set the scene, develop the characters, build on the plot and then bring it all home. The same applies to his dinner parties, and everything is planned to the detail well in advance. In essence, his guests are walking through his story and leave the evening with a juicy version of their own to tell. Along with delicious food, this is how and why his party invitations are so coveted.

A similar process can and should occur in the dental practice. Often the stories are a flare for the dramatic. A crisis occurs. The patient seeks help, and a heroine or hero miraculously appears. A battle or conflict ensues. The hero prevails, and the patient is overjoyed and relieved that the issue is resolved.

Understand that the communication used along the patient's journey will dictate what story they tell about their experience at your office.

An exercise we have found to be effective is dissecting personal experiences with various customer service agents. Try thinking back to a time you had a problem with your car. What language was used? What emotion was conveyed? Were you reassured that they would help you or were you met with a statement of how busy they are? Were the words, I'm not sure when we can... used?

Now think back to an exceptional experience. How were the language and attitude different? How did you feel when the conversation ended?

Do This

-Practice scripting compassionate and honest responses for the most common requests

-Ensure the patient hears and feels your desire to help solve their problem

-We are all busy, but try not to let that mentality cause you to rush through conversations

Need some help? Try this guide for your Dental Practice

Brain On

Fueling The Brain For Growth

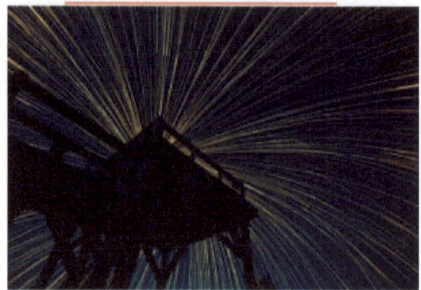

BRAIN ON

DENTAL PRACTICE RESOURCE GROUP

The option is to step forward into growth or remain stagnant and slide behind into safety. This is a variation of Abraham Maslow's famous quote, and it holds important value for everyone seeking to make an impact on the world.

Education is a key differentiator and creating an environment reward effort creates not only intelligently motivated team members but also fosters happiness and satisfaction. Increasing knowledge increases value and creating the spark of interest in learning and raise the level of your staff's abilities.

Partner with everyone in the practice and commit to learning and a growth mindset. I have found that once the process starts it remains in perpetual motion as the excitement of learning and sharing is contagious. This happened recently as one of our best assistants started a hygiene program and excited to finish and rejoin the practice.

Foster growth and look for continuing education opportunities that support the growth of the team member as well as the practice.

Do This:

-Make a personal commitment to learning beyond the minimum required by your state board
-Support your team and encourage self-directed learning
-Provide opportunities to learn as an office
-Build teamwork and camaraderie by attending CE meetings together

What is your favorite activity for learning and growing as a team?

photo credit: jimmy-musto

Getting To Go

Guide Your Flock - Getting To Confident Proficiency

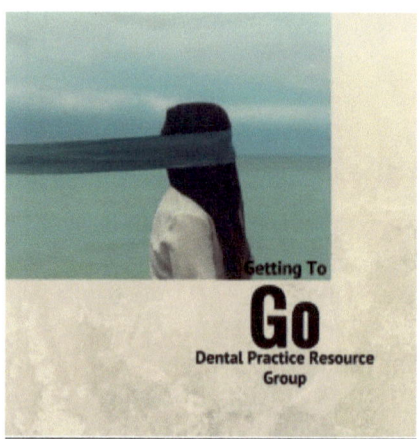

At some point in all lives, we are all new.

New school.

New partner.

New job.

Although labeled as exciting, a certain degree of anxiety is inevitable. Nowhere is this more evident than in the high stakes arena of health care. The spotlight is always on, and we often practice in a fishbowl with others peering down and analyzing our actions.

The learning curve of joining a new dental practice is steep and can be arduous, but an elegant solution exists.

Call it what you like, teammate, buddy or mentor, the result is the same. By pairing up new members with an experienced teammate, a smooth transition is created and anxieties quelled in the process.

Having someone who knows the ropes can make a huge impact on the effectiveness of new hires. Too often a person is hired and rushed through an orientation and then turned loose with the anticipation of being a competent, fully-functioning team member.

The pace in most dental practices is brisk, and room turnovers are prompt and efficient. We have a schedule to keep and want to deliver a consistently amazing experience for all patients.

A brief pause is warranted, and a closer look is needed to understand the futility of most orientation programs. Is it reasonable to expect someone to join the team, learn the office policies and culture, master the nuances of dental software, digital equipment, and patient preferences in a matter of one or two weeks? Have you ever had a new hire quit within a few months? How much time, effort and expense did that waste?

Our approach attempts to make the orientation process a bit gentler. Each new hire has already been assigned a buddy/mentor before coming onboard. Most of our best candidates go through a working interview to assess their ability to provide service to our patients in a caring manner. This also lets the mentor determine if they are someone they would like to work with and call a team member. Observing these interactions helps us make more intelligent hiring decisions.

After hire, they work one: one for two to three weeks to ensure they have mastered the essentials of the practice. Then the mentor steps back and observes from a distance but is ready to step in during moments of confusion, panic or crisis. This process ensures the new team member feels supported in their role. We have found their productivity and ability to contribute to the practice quickly reaches the level of other team members.

The mentor-buddy period formally ends with an interview. This allows both sides to express opinions and ideas about the process, resolve questions, and transitions the new staffer into a fully vested member of our team. The mentor-buddy relationship continues, and both sides agree to a door-always-open policy to ensure any issues are promptly addressed.

Do This:

-After selecting the best candidate(s), bring them back and let them interact with the patients

-Assign a buddy or mentor from day 1 to facilitate the orientation and transition process

-Understand that a job transition often takes longer than anticipated

-Don't release the lamb to the wolves without ensuring all new hires are fully supported in every capacity required to ensure effectiveness

Photo credit: Oscar Keys

Hit Reset

Every Day is a New Day

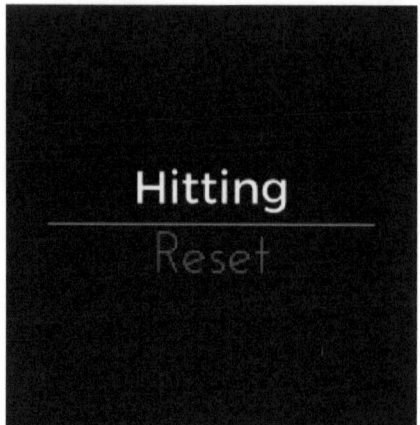

To a patient, you are only as good as your last visit.

Every day is a new day and the clock resets to zero. Patients keep score and remember both good and bad experiences.

As health care professionals, we are blessed with the opportunity to begin anew with every patient encounter. Starting over allows us to build upon an already excellent reputation. Accept the challenge and don't rest on your laurels.

All of us experience bad days and unsatisfactory patient encounters. It is a part of the practice. Sometimes it's due to a bad night's sleep or feeling under the weather. Other times the explanation is harder to decipher, but try to tease out the reason. Then resolve to hit reset and start fresh with the next patient or next day.

●

Do This:

Hit reset and start every day fresh

Understand that we are only as good as our last patient or procedure

Every day is an opportunity to reach for perfection

Earn your excellent reputation with every patient interaction

Give patients a reason to sing your praises

Focus On One

Be Open

Open or Closed?

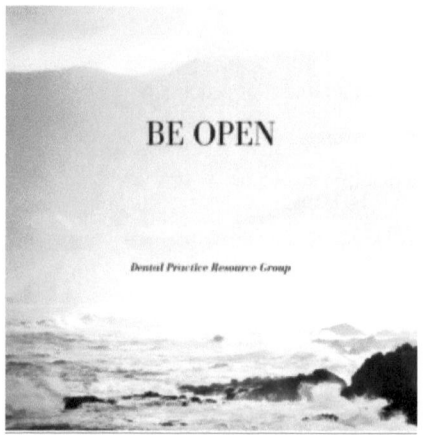

Consider how you would typically respond to these two questions:

1) How are you today?

2) What is the one thing that if you accomplished it today, would make all the difference and why?

The first question is met with a one or two-word response, and little information is gained from that exchange.

The second question piques interest and should generate a more robust result. It also fosters an ongoing dialogue that allows a deeper connection.

In today's busy world, we are quick to get off the phone, hurry to wrap up conversations, and blurt out rapid-fire answers so we can get on our way or back to what we were doing.

Take a moment and consider who you feel when rushed to get off a call. How many times has another question popped into your head as soon as you hung up? Add a bit of anxiety or stress and now envision how a patient feels when their concerns are hurried through or put off with curt answers.

Rephrasing scripted questions provides patients an opportunity to openly share concerns or questions. The habit of asking closed-ended questions is tough to break, but the reward to shifting to open-ended questions combined with a caring and curious attitude creates the type of dental experience we all crave. Questions are answered fully; information exchanged and education provided leaving the patient satisfied and more likely to accept treatment.

Consider the following:

What are you here for today? vs. What concerns or questions can I solve for you today?

The second drives the conversation towards solving the real concern of the patient. Sure, they may be here for a simple filling, but probing deeper you might be surprised to learn that they have symptoms of sleep apnea and may benefit from an oral appliance or referral for a sleep study. One of our dentists has completed advanced training in dental sleep medicine and receives frequent praise for improving patients' lives and health.

Are you ready to do this procedure? vs. How do you think this will change your smile and do you have any concerns before proceeding?

The first question begets a simple "yes" answer. The other opens up dialogue for larger issues. A simple composite filling may be all that was offered, but perhaps the patient desires a complete anterior makeover since her best friend has a beautiful smile thanks to her dentist's veneer work. If you don't probe deeper, you can't solve the larger issue lurking under the surface.

Do you want to accept this treatment plan? vs. What would keep you from moving forward with improving your smile today?

Often more than one decision maker is involved, and it may not be the patient sitting in your chair. Uncovering who makes the final determination or what barriers to acceptance exist can help you solve their concerns. Ever heard "I didn't know you offered Care Credit or payment plans for this type of cosmetic work"? Don't write off a "No" as the final answer when the topic is broached with a closed-ended Yes/No question. Give patients the opportunity to share the reasoning behind their choices.

Do This:

- Encourage dialogue by using open-ended questions
- Be aware of body language and voice tonality
- Rephrase common issues:

  -What concerns or questions can I solve for you   today?

  -How do you think this will change your smile and do you have any concerns before proceeding?

  -What would keep you from moving forward with improving your smile today?

Bend Reality

You Have The Power To Bend Reality

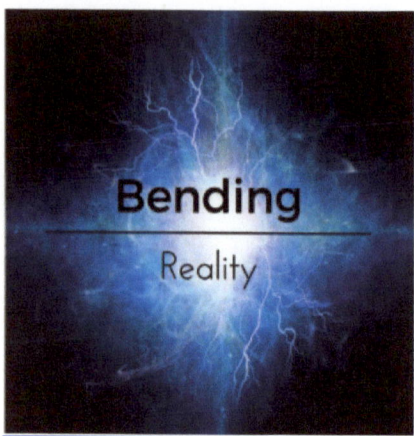

Wouldn't it be cool if you could bend reality and create the world as you desire?

You may not have super powers, but you and your team have the ability to shape and even bend the perception of your patients.

By crafting the initial exposure to your practice, you can develop the patient's reality and impression of your office. It is as simple as ensuring that their first impression is amazing. Don't let this opportunity slip by; it will never come around again. There is only one chance to make a first impression.

I am a realist and understand how busy and chaotic a typical day is in a dental practice. That said, having a team that performs professionally on a consistent basis will set your office apart. It takes practice and diligence to smile when the proverbial crap is hitting the fan.

Try approaching things from an anxious or nervous patient's perspective. Would you rather be met with a warm greeting and friendly, inviting smile or a hurried utterance of "Take a seat, and I'll be with you when I get a second"?

Even when a difficult patient opens the office door and steps towards the front desk, our team has adopted the strategy of greeting everyone as if a best friend just walked in the door.

Be conscious of body language and facial expressions. Most new patients see the front desk staff as the face of the practice and make assumptions about how the experience will go based on their first 30 seconds inside your office. When the front desk staff has a permanent scowl or furrowed brow, the tone is set, and patients may adopt this same attitude.

I took my child to a specialist's office this morning for an initial consult. The front desk receptionist sat facing the door and was rather attractive. She was well-dressed and appeared professional. Despite standing directly in front of her, she didn't offer a greeting or bother to look up from her computer. I had to walk around the desk and approach a different staff member who was much friendlier and offered a smile, a warm welcome, and made sure we were comfortable while waiting. Had she not been there, I have no idea what the other staffer would have done to acknowledge our presence. Even a simple smile or wave would have been better than being ignored.

No one likes to be ignored or making patients feel like they are intruding on a private party creates a first impression that is damaging to the practice.

Do This:
- Greet every patient in a positive manner
- Set the tone and ensure patients are comfortable while waiting
- Be conscious of body language and facial expressions
- Assess the patient's mood based on cues and adjust your greeting on an individual basis
-

Have It Your Way

Script without the script

Miscommunication leads to errors. Miscommunication leads to accidents. Misinterpretation results in wrong decisions.

In a perfect world, our patients would speak the same language we do. You and I both know that is just a fantasy, but adapting to how each patient communicates is crucial for avoiding errors, problems, and unhappy patients.

Learn to interpret their individual communication style. It takes experience and practice, but the effort clearly pays off.

It is important to remember that patients have their own agenda and desires. While you may want to restore anteriorly and replace a crown, they may be focused on a tuition bill for their college freshman or wondering if an implant may be a better option.

Without an honest and upfront discussion, your team will never know what drives their acceptance or rejection of your treatment plan. Pay attention to subtle cues and body language. Established patients often become like family and picking up on subtle signs becomes easier, but don't be afraid to ask. Patients often appreciate a caring gesture or understanding ear.

Do This:

- Recognize that a patient has their agenda and will not always share it without being asked

   Educate without pushing
- Work to understand individual patient needs and deliver on that

Not For Everyone

The temptation to satisfy and be liked is innate to our human psyche.

We want to be everything for everybody at times. Unfortunately, this leads to an equilibration point of mediocrity. The fruit of this sort of labor is to be average.

Since you are reading this, I feel safe in assuming you want something else for yourself and your dental practice.

Adjust The Mark

Consider the result of setting lofty goals and missing them. The result produced is often much greater than if safe or easily obtainable goals are chosen.

When a person aims high and misses, so what. This is not failure. Try reframing the interpretation of what happened.

It wasn't failure; a result was produced. In this scenario, that result is often what makes the difference between a memorable/amazing experience and a "just average" outcome.

Do This:

- Reframe expectations and goals

- Accept missing the mark

- Erase "failure" and replace it with "result"

- Aim for outliers & the mean will sort itself

The One In The Middle

Do More Than The Middle

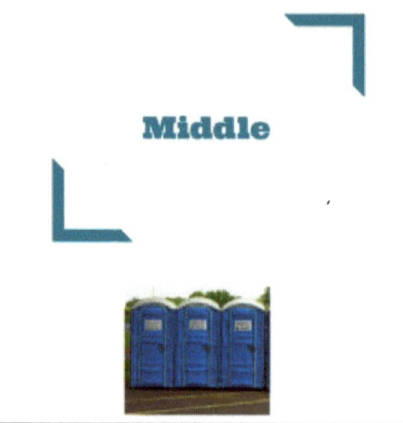

Delivering average care or creating an average experience does nothing to help a business. The following story shares a recent experience to illustrate this point.

Typically when I go to the grocery store, I'm in a hurry. I want to get in and out as fast as possible.

Recently, I got to the checkout and realized I forgot the two specific items my wife requested. I hurried back to where I thought the items were located but had not luck. Fortunately, three employees were standing nearby in a conversation.

As I approached, one turned to me and stared blankly when I asked for help finding two items. The other kept talking to the third with his back to me. Noticing I needed help, the third employee offered to show me exactly where I needed to go. The first employee jumped in stating that aisle 6 is probably right. Needless to say, I didn't have a clue where aisle 6 was. Thirty seconds later, with the help of the third employee, I was on my way through checkout with the mission complete.

This simple example plays out in healthcare settings every day. Think about your practice and how your team assists patients. Do new patients get a tour? If someone asks to use a bathroom, does your team show them or just point down the hall? If a problem such as spilled coffee on the waiting room floor is reported, do staff jump to action or say they will get to it when they can?

Do This:
- Go the extra mile and make everything easy for patients
- Treat them like guests in your home
- Be cognizant of a patient's expression that suggests they need help or have a problem

Final Performance

How Are You Performing?

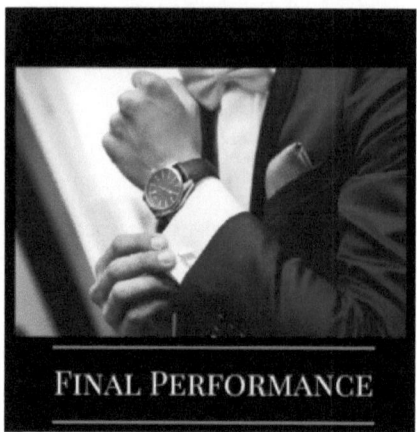

Life as a dental professional means that you are always on stage. Front and center with the spotlight directed on you.

Each performance must be delivered with precision, passion and enthusiasm. Perform as if you're giving the show of your career.

Health care is a lot like sports. When you are suited up and step on the field, it's "go time." Patients expect that you will show up to play every day and give it your all.

Be a Total Professional

We all have personal lives, nights of poor sleep, and other baggage that must be managed. Checking that stuff before you deliver care and focusing on "now" is essential. Although it may be tempting to share your woes with patients, they are there for themselves. Don't shift focus off their needs or cares to lament about your troubles. Catharsis is best reserved for another time and setting.

Do This:

- • Commit to pleasing and delivering the "show" of your life
- • Be ready to perform and show up prepared to deliver
- • Behave is if you are the key actor in a sold out show
- • Make today better than yesterday and tomorrow better than today
- • Strive to raise the level of your game - set new standard
- • Treat every day like it's the last

Means Not Ends

Why Focus On Means

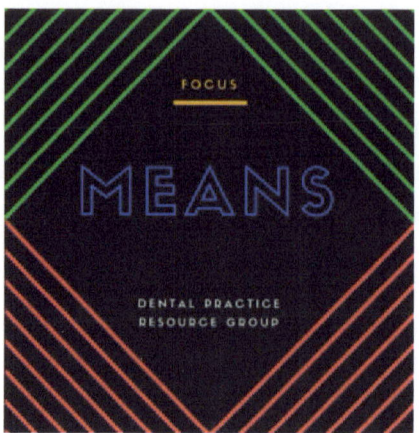

What is the ultimate goal in your dental practice?

Narrow down that running list in your head to the one overriding all-encompassing goal.

What is it? Write it down. One sentence or less.

Is it to?

-Make money

-Occupy your time

-Get you out of the house

-Stimulate your mind

-Make patients happy and grow personally and professionally

It's All About The Means

When your focus lies on the end goal, the journey loses its magic. What happens when the goal is reached? The celebration is followed by a sense of sadness or emptiness.

The best part of any experience is the journey. Sure victory is sweet and reaching the summit is cool, but then what? Relentless focus on a single goal, often a number, creates a culture driven by dollar signs that ignores the journey.

This chapter is not intended to be Pollyanna in principle but bring attention back to "why." Why you became a dentist or dental specialist.

Focusing on deploying all your skills and talents to solve a patient's problem and improve their oral health creates value beyond a number.

Focusing on the means equals a great dental experience combined with excellent care creating happy patients who accept treatment plans and grow your practice's income and patient load.

A case in point, several years ago we refitted the office with new computers. During due diligence, two experts were consulted, and it became apparent that their goals were completely different. The first was pushing hard for a sale and quick close. The second gushed enthusiasm for technology and took the time to understand our specific needs. In the end, he talked us out of a more expensive package and delivered precisely what we needed. We have been back several times to purchase additional gear, and his focus on the means has given him a customer for life.

Do This:

- Listen and understand patient needs as it's easier to keep existing than recruit new ones
- Focus on the means and avoid pushing for the sale - when patients know you care, everyone wins
- Care for patients' human needs and seize the opportunity to make their journey amazing

Ask Better Questions

Ask Better Questions

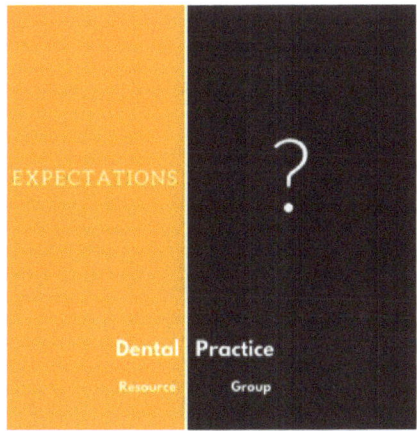

The key to a better life is asking better questions. The key to optimizing patient expectations and outcomes is to make sure they are asking the right questions.

Take the following example:

Patient: How much will this big filling cost?

Staff: With insurance, about $75 for a composite or tooth-colored filling.

Patient: Geez. Well, o.k. Let's do that at the next appointment.

Staff: Great. We look forward to seeing you soon.

How often does a conversation similar to this play out in your dental practice? What could be going wrong with this exchange?

The job as a dental professional is to make sure patients have all the information to make intelligent healthcare decisions. This scenario leaves a lot out.

Take the initiative and help patients see the long term cost of decisions made today. In this instance, the large filling has a real potential of failing and the tooth will need more expensive treatment - root canal, crown, extraction, bridge or even an implant. We are all aware of how expensive anything related to health is, but make sure your patients see the full impact of their decisions. Letting cost be the only factor misses the mark of providing amazing dental care.

By educating patients, they will learn to ask or at least understand better questions such as:
-What's the long-term consequence of putting this procedure off for 6 months to a year?
-If the filling fails, what is the next step and how much does it cost?
-Will ignoring this cause me to lose the tooth later?
-What options are there for paying for the best care for my tooth?

Patients often have a different timeline in mind than you do.
Keep the conversation flowing and make sure they have a solid understanding of when the treatment should be completed. Soon to you very likely means something entirely different to them.

Keep Going

Don't be afraid to ask questions after answering theirs. By probing deeper, you ensure patients are getting what they need vs. minimal care.

If a patient seems to be making a choice that will compromise their oral health, try rephrasing the questions.

-In a perfect world, what treatment would you like to do?

-Is there a particular part of what we proposed to do that makes you uncomfortable?

-I know your treatment plan is complex, is there anything you'd like me to go over again?

Do This:

- Maintain a sense of curiosity to understand patient decisions
- Don't abandon patients - dentistry can be complicated and make sure they know their options and the best option
- Bridge the gap between what they want vs. need
- Ask questions and help the patient understand their care
- Follow up questions can reveal hidden concerns
-

Finding Yes

Why No Means Yes

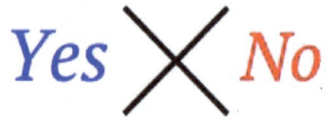

Patients expect you to solve their problems. They want and need you to find the yes.

No is a powerful word and can shut people down quickly. Think back to childhood and how you felt when a parent replied "No" to your request, seemingly before you even finished the sentence. How did it make you feel?

Patients are often anxious, rushed or in pain. Hearing "no'" along with subtle negative body language or tone, causes the atmosphere to deteriorate further.

Instead of uttering a quick "No" to difficult requests, one option is to rephrase it.

-Let me find something that works for you and gives the dentist enough time to solve your problem

-I understand your situation. Let's work and see how to work around it.

-Instead of, "No, we can't see you today," substitute "The schedule is completely full today, and we want to make it a priority to see you tomorrow. Can that work with your schedule?"

Do This:

- Find a way to say, "Yes!"
- Remove "No" as much as possible during conversations with patients
- Working in a dental practice is stressful and busy, but don't let negative body language and tone result in "No," being the default response to patient questions
-

Selling Trust

Educate, Empower and Sell Through Trust

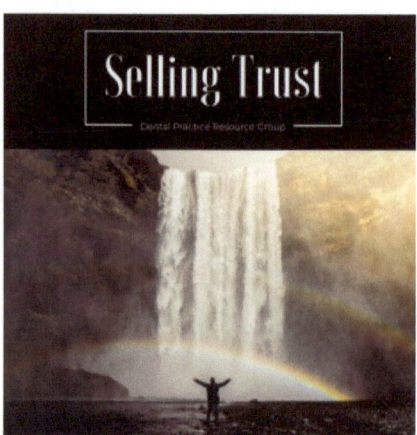

Although most who work in healthcare view themselves as professional healers, they often have difficulty accepting and trusting their role as a salesperson.

Patients are customers and not showing them the goods is doing them a disservice.

Replace the discomfort of selling with a mindset of educating. Informed patients are more likely to make the best choice for their unique needs.

Your patients trust your years of experience and expertise. Resist the temptation to prejudge whether or not someone will accept a more expensive treatment option or cosmetic procedure. Studies are clear that healthcare providers are often wrong when guessing patient expectations.

The bottom line is that by upselling a better treatment, both your patient and practice win.

Common Situation

A patient is unhappy with their smile. The hygienist recommends whitening and the dentist suggests anterior composites on #8 and 9. The patient isn't interested in either option. Both the dentist and hygienist shrug it off and consider the issue dead. In reality, this patient is interested in Invisalign, but doesn't think she is a candidate and is not at all interested in traditional orthodontia. If no one bothers to ask what her true needs or desires are, solving them becomes infinitely more challenging.

Team Sport

Take a moment and survey your staff on how often a patient asks for more information as soon as the dentist steps away from the chair. Patients are complex emotional machines and may hold back questions out of fear of looking silly or asking a "dumb" question. This is just human nature. Empower your team to promote and sell services. For example, a patient asks about chairside whitening during a hygiene exam. The dentist shares the relevant information, comments on the upcoming wedding of the patient's daughter and wraps up that portion of the visit. The hygienist then introduces

Invisalign as a way to further enhance the patient's smile and that it can fit in her timeline before the wedding day.

Do This:

- Ask questions so you can make better suggestions to enhance the patient's care
- Don't assume you can predict patients' decisions
- Use education and teach the patient about their options and empower them to make better decisions
- Don't be afraid to sell - it's the lifeblood of growing your practice

photo credit: Jared Erondu

Confirming Emotion

The Last Emotion

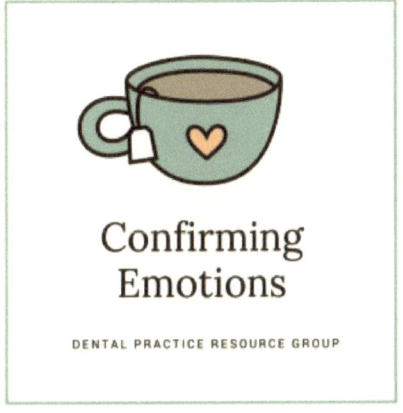

Although a first impression is vital, it's not the only part of the equation. The last few minutes of every appointment provides a wealth of opportunity. Take advantage of solidifying the amazing experience your team has just delivered. Give them a reason to think of your practice in the kindest terms.

A few options our team uses:

-Help an elderly patient to their car

-Send home a small container of Ben & Jerry's for all extraction patients

-Thank them for coming in today

-Walk them up and share a simple smile before they leave

The last few moments are also an opportunity to address and correct any shortcomings. Offer an apology for a late start and make sure the patient understands that you value their time. Use positive phrases powered by a caring and concerned attitude. We have a stack of coffee cards to several local shops and bistros so the patient can pick. This simple gesture goes a long way to leaving a lasting impression, even if there were some stumbling blocks along the patient's journey through the visit.

Do This:

- Consider the comfort of every patient
- Offer a warm neck wrap or blanket
- End with a positive moment to overcome any misadventures
- Give them a reason to love your practice

Child's Play

Easy Peasey

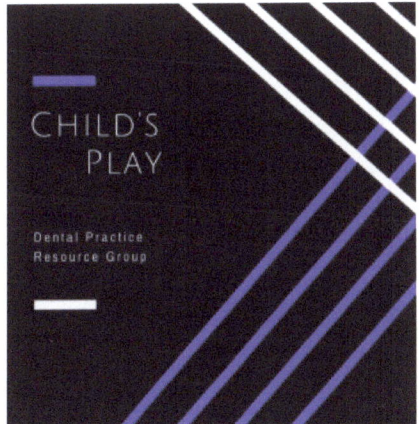

Think back to when you mastered riding a bike. The first few tries were likely harrowing and full of more than a few crashes. Quickly you learned to master the skills to navigate around and over a variety of obstacles. The unexpected dip in the road or wrong turn will undoubtedly cause upset or anger, but you keep going and reap the glory of wind wiping through your hair as you carve your way through new adventures.

It's easy to become lulled into a routine when everything seems to be humming along smoothly. Patients are happy; the team is working efficiently; you are unstoppable. Then you hit a large pothole and are derailed. The patient is mad, and their spouse is angry. The patient is crying, and the hovering mother is shrieking that you are hurting her child. It happens.

Respond to these situations by stepping back and using a simple formula to restore order and solve any lapses in communication with the patient.

1) Step Back

When the conversation is headed off course, ask for a time out or moment to think about the issue. Having a patient yelling in your face in the waiting room is detrimental to all involved. Usher them into a consult room, if possible. If they are in a hurry and the matter is not immediately solvable, ask them for a specific time to reconnect to resolve their concerns.

2) Take A Breath

Now that you have stepped back take a moment to cool down. Resist the temptation to dwell on the drama.

Distract yourself by taking on a new task. Let the stress hormones clear and let your mind relax.

3) Learning Opportunity

Approach analysis from the patient's point of view. What happened or failed to happen? How could you have approached this issue differently? What is the best possible outcome for this problem? Solving problems often requires asking better questions.

4) Team Up

       Incident debriefing is valuable in crisis situations. Use this opportunity to share this event with other team members. Brainstorm solutions that are unique to this patient. Several other staff have likely interacted with them and can offer insight on peculiarities in conversation style or attitude. Was the patient just having a bad day, did something catastrophic happen in their life or are they just a difficult person?

Knowing this information completely reframes the situation and can result in a solution readily appearing.

Do This:

- Step back when situations are spiraling out of control
- Consult your team for insight and options
- Admit when you're wrong and fix it quickly
- Resist the temptation to internalize and argue

Own Everything

You Must Own It

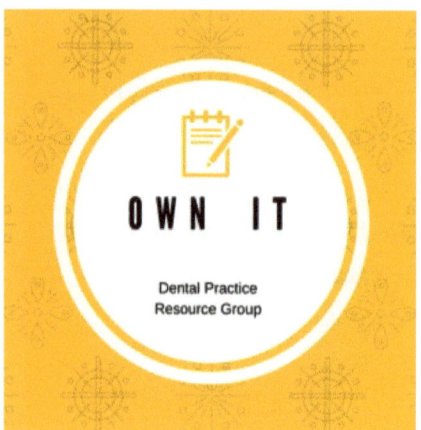

We can decide to accept responsibility or make excuses. The choice should be simple, but human emotion makes it complicated.

Taking personal responsibility for the experiences of our patients and owning the entire process is a powerful way to shift the mindset of individuals and culture of a practice. Patients will quickly realize that your team is on their side.

You are what stands between the patient and their happiness and satisfaction with the services you deliver. Accepting both the good and bad outcomes and expressing your concern fosters a strong bond between the patient and your practice.

While we all know dentistry is part art and part science, patients don't often see it that way. In their mind, an extraction should be a cookbook procedure and nothing should go wrong. Some will even draw the analogy to getting their car oil changed. They want prompt service, no hassles, and a consistent result. Don't fault them for their beliefs, even though we as healthcare professionals know the body doesn't always cooperate with our treatment and procedures.

During residency training, we were required to keep a patient log and call back at least 10% of our patients every month. At the time, this practice was painful and seemed burdensome, the result was nothing short of incredible. We received feedback on our procedures, recognized mistakes, provided reassurance and education to the patients and improved rapport.

Carrying this habit forward is a simple, yet valuable way to convey an attitude of ownership to our patients' happiness. Our staff calls patients as well, but when one of our dentists or oral surgeons makes the call, patients take notice.

These follow-up calls are an opportunity to troubleshoot problems. More than one potential disaster was averted after our dentist learned of unusual facial swelling or severe pain under the tongue. As you know, patients don't always follow instructions or take their antibiotics as prescribed.

Patients quickly learn that your care is amazing at the chairside <u>and</u> on the follow-through. Delivering care at a higher level shows accountability and immediately creates a strong bond between patients and your practice.

Do This

- Own everything completely - the good and bad
- The entire team adopts an attitude of accountability
- Call back patients and give them support and respect
- Solve the patient's problem(s)

Defuse The Wrong

Defusing The Wrong

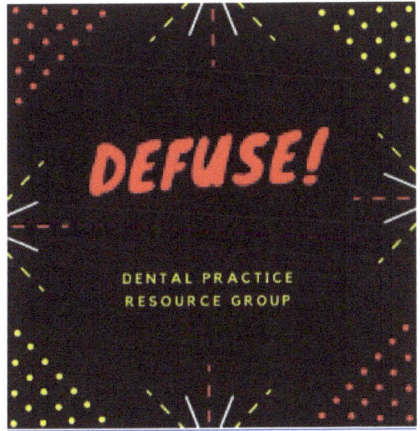

For pride is spiritual cancer: it eats up every possibility of love, or contentment or even common sense.

-C.S. Lewis

Pride is a powerful emotion and arguing leads to anger and creates distance between you and the patient.

Although one doesn't have to agree with every customer-patient, they do deserve respect. Acting like mistakes are never made and refusing to take any part in owning the problem increases the difficulty and stress of solving a patient issue.

This is not promoting the false notion that the patient (customer) is always right. Even when you know they are wrong; respect is still required if you want to keep them as a patient. Resist the temptation to escalate the situation just to prove your point.

People hate being proven wrong. Rubbing their face in it by pontificating and barraging them with ten reasons why they are wrong will do little to solve the core problem.

While difficult, try not to take their comments and finger-pointing personally. Often fear or worry are at the heart of their statements. Take a moment and look at the situation as if you were their best friend or significant other. How would you feel about the situation? This can often provide an avenue to begin solving their problem.

Our practice utilizes an automated reminder system and is driven by patient preferences. After scheduling an appointment, the system will send them an email, a text or a phone call. Some patients choose all three options and the system seamlessly delivers. We accept that technological glitches can occur, cell phone signals can be poor or calls dropped, but overall the system is highly reliable.

On occasion, a patient will show up on the wrong day or time and emphatically state they have an appointment. Our front desk staff is trained not to argue or prove the patient wrong' but to attempt to solve the problem. Options are offered, gaps in the day are found to accommodate when possible and the staff work to resolve the problem. Respect for the patient remains the top priority. Remaining caring, understanding and flexible reassures the patient that our practice values them. Patients often come away feeling satisfied even if they were not seen that day.

Do This:

- Respect the patient and their opinion
- Accept the difference between facts and patient perceptions
- Solve the problem

Restoring Grace

Graceful Disagreements

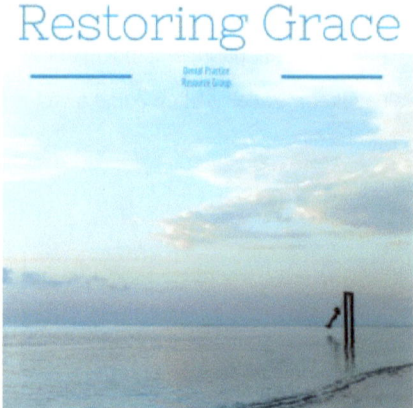

Human nature often compels us to attempt to save face. Our quick reaction is to argue and work passionately with the goal of coercing the other person into seeing things our way.

The challenge is to remember what profession you chose. You are not a lawyer. Putting the patient at the center of everything provides clear direction on where all actions must be aligned. In any disagreement, the goal must be to recover the respect and trust of the patient. That is if you want to keep them as a patient.

Showing your true colors and putting personal feelings aside while respecting your team and the patient goes a long way to solving an issue. Apologize when needed and do it without grudge. We are not in 3rd grade anymore. We are the consummate professional.

Back up words with action. Not every solution will be readily apparent, but even temporizing a solution shows the patient that you are vested in their happiness. This will provide time until an acceptable permanent resolution is found. The final answer will be more than just a quick fix. It must restore trust and confidence in the practice and yourself.

Try doing the unexpected. When a problem surfaces, some patients show up expecting a fight and the adrenaline is surging from the moment of go. This is your opportunity to show them some magic. Use empathy and work to understand how they are feeling and know that some confusion likely exists. Perhaps they didn't understand the insurance code or their copay. Take a moment to calmly go over the treatment plan estimates they agreed upon. Time has a way of clouding memory and doing so with a calm and polite voice often diffuses the situation. Help them to understand how their bill was created and walk them through what procedures were completed. Your explanation will guide them to realizing the value of your services.

While every patient is different, many common scenarios occur on a frequent basis. Consider the following:
-Why is my bill so much
-I didn't agree to this charge
-I don't understand why "you" charged me for x,y and z
-Why do I have a copay
-I don't think a crown should cost so much. What are you going to do to help me?

-Your office just wants to make lots of money

-I bet the dentist is driving that fancy car I saw out front

Use the power of your team to create thoughtful responses to these and other difficult situations and comments. Leaving people to think on the fly and respond off the cuff often fails to generate thoughtful responses that respect the patient, even when they are wrong.

Do This:

Show them you have a sense of urgency to help solve their problem

Create scenarios and scripts to guide your team

Empower your team to solve the problems

Photo credit: Azrul Aziz

Your Time, My Time

Managing Expectations

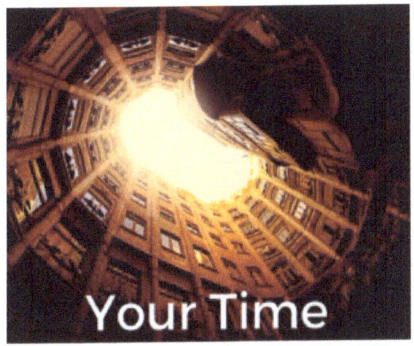

Dental Practice Resource Group

I was in a bit of a hurry and hustled in to get the oil changed at my local dealer. They are usually pretty quick, and I'm in and out in 30 minutes. The parking lot was empty, and the waiting room was deserted. I was confident that I'd be headed down the road shortly.

As the clock spun by, I began to fidget. After 45 minutes, I inquired at the desk and was told it was almost done. After another 30 minutes, I was angry. The manager came out and explained there had been a lift malfunction, and an employee was badly injured. He apologized for the delay, and I felt deflated.

As I sat and waited some more, I still felt a bit on edge. Why hadn't someone advised the now full waiting room on why things were taking longer than usual. Even just a quick one sentence explanation would have diffused the rising frustration felt by us as customers.

Minutes Matter

Healthcare visits often generate anxiety and expectation. Keeping patients waiting without explanation gives the impression that their time is not valued.

The Disney theme parks have this down to a science. When in line, visitors know how long their wait will be and are entertained, or at least distracted, while they wait.

Urgent care centers have adopted a similar patient-centered time focus with great success. Patients can see in real time online what the anticipated wait is at various clinics. Armed with this information lets them choose where they want to be seen.

Respect and honor your patients time. Keep them updated and happy while they wait. Patients understand or care that your extraction was difficult and the day unfolded because your first two patients were late. They only care about themselves and their time. Accept this reality.

Your job is to exceed their expectations if you want to create an amazing experience and grow. Provide honest answers and be realistic. Don't set your practice up for failure by over promising and under delivering. It needs to be the other way around.

Distract Them

Give the patient something to do while waiting. Having a sterile silent waiting room scares patients away. Create engaging opportunities and keep magazines current. Think about how you feel when your doctor's office has three-year-old copies of Sports Illustrated or Home and Garden lying about. Let them know you care about their comfort and happiness.

Our office quietly plays National Geographic videos in the waiting room suitable for any age. Magazines are refreshed monthly, and options for different interests are available. We periodically poll our patients about which they prefer to read. We also have a free book box where patients and staff supply books for the taking. A children's corner keeps the little ones engaged and distracted. We also have educational activities and monthly contests where patients can win prizes.

Do This:

Treat patients' time like it is your own

Provide honest answers and work to exceed expectations

Update and apologize when needed

Create an engaging and entertaining waiting room

Photo credit: alexandre-perotto

Relationship Poison

Words Kill

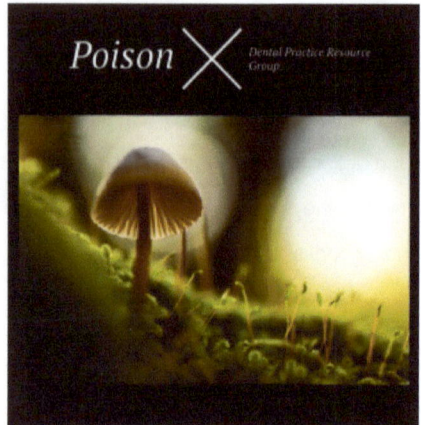

Words kill, words give life; they're either poison or fruit - you choose
Proverbs 18:21

Solving patient problems requires flexibility and patience. Just think back to the last time you called a customer service department and how did that person make you feel? Was your time valued and your issue taken seriously? Were you given a workable solution or put off or told to try back later when so and so was back from vacation?

Certain phrases that immediately raise patients blood pressure and create doubt that your practice is any different than then next down the road.

Consider the following responses and how do they make you feel like as patient?

-I don't have anything to do with that. Sorry, you'll have to call back.

-We never do that sort of thing. You'll have to have multiple appointments.

-I can't help you with that and the person who can isn't here right now.

All of these responses let the patient know that they wasted time and effort trying to solve their problem. It also signals resistance from the dental practice staff. None of these phrases provide any inkling that the patient is valued.

Previous chapters have discussed empowering your team to be flexible in solving patient problems. Even temporary solutions ensure the patients feels understood and appreciated.

Patients direct all questions and concerns at the front desk staff and want quick answers, but the final decision often lies with the dentist, hygienist or office manager. Ensure that the patient knows their concern or complaint was heard. Register understanding and respect and let them know it will be handled. Tell them what action will be taken to resolve their problem. Tell them to feel free to call you with questions and that an update will be forthcoming with an answer.

Patients have their agendas and aren't always forthcoming about why they want what they want. An unusual request may boil down to an impending move, layoff or loss of insurance. Remember the asking better questions discussion? Probing a bit deeper often reveals the real motivation and helps the team create an appropriate response.

Here is a typical scenario in our office:
A patient calls and wants to see hygiene, complete a treatment plan for an extraction and composite restoration in another quadrant and have her two children seen in

hygiene at the same visit. Oh, and she needs the appointment to be at 4:30 due to a new job. She also wants to sit down with the office manager and discuss her bill.

Our staff listens intently and lets her know that she wants to make this all happen. The hygienists are busy with patients, but she tells the patient she will have an answer and appointment date within the hour and asks for a good number to call the patient back.

There is a lot going on in this one phone call. While tempting to just tell the patient the last hygiene appointment is at 4:30 and she will have to reschedule her kids another day, the staff takes a moment to discuss it with the hygiene department and find a workable solution. She messages the dentist in Slack and makes a note to herself to follow up with the patient.

Do This:
Listen with empathy and reiterate a desire to help
Bring the patient closer to an answer even if you can't solve it immediately
Track, delegate, and follow-up
Find a tool or system that works for your office (Slack, Trello, etc)

photo credit: manuel-barroso-parejo

Now

Focus on Now

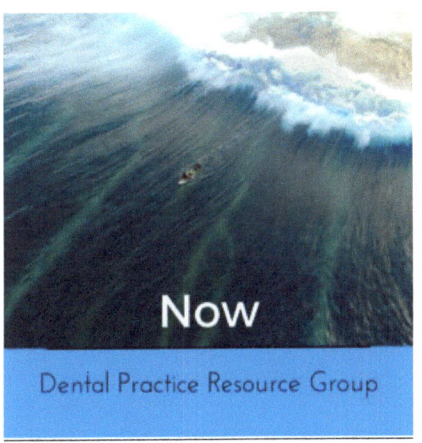

This book has a bit of philosophy wrapped up in the strategies shared so far. This quote has substantial application in how a dental practice interacts with its patients:

Realize that the present moment is all you ever have.

-Eckhart Tolle

In a typical day in any dental practice anywhere in the world it's easy to be sucked into the swirling vortex of hell. Patients everywhere, hygiene checks, equipment problems, phone calls, product reps, emergencies, rushing to get out the door to pick up kids are the norm. Never mind finding a bit of time to scarf down food or use the bathroom.

We are only human and deserve to treat ourselves with compassion and understanding. Now, this moment, is all anyone is ever guaranteed.

The same applies to interactions with patients, especially new ones. Resist the temptation to rush ahead to future. Hold off on envisioning what procedures they need and the added production.

Focus on now. How are you showing up? What kind of interaction is taking place? Does the patient see you and your staff as caring, attentive and interested in their complete well-being or do they feel like a commodity or number to be quickly shuffled into the funnel of appointments and procedures.

Pause and take just a brief moment to consider how you want them to describe the practice and you in particular. What description and emotion do you want to be used?

Seize this moment to create the amazing experience every patient desires. Help the patient perceive you as the best answer to their dental health problems.

Do This:
Pause and take a moment before rapidly plowing ahead with a new patient visit
Focus on now and create the type of experience you would want as a new patient
Every time a patient is in contact with any aspect of your practice, they are forming an opinion
Ensure that what you are doing now fosters positive emotion and encourages the patient to return again

Photo Credit: ishan-seefromthesky

Beyond Ordinary

Own The Race Track

Control The Course, Own The Result

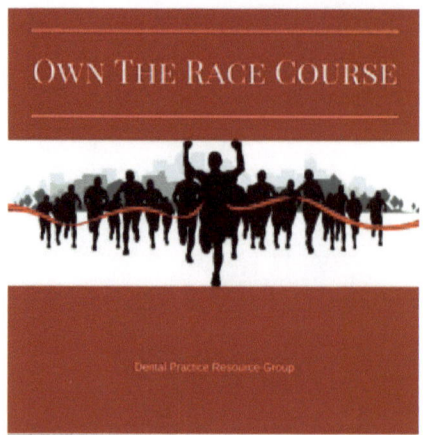

<u>Focus on the one thing you do really well.</u>

-James Schramko (internet marketing billionaire)

One can decide to do everything or do something. It is that decision that produces a moment of mediocrity or a moment of greatness. The beauty lies in the fact that you get to decide.

While patients expect a general degree of competency across the dental sphere, not many will know the significance of a 1 mm margin or why a particular material choice makes all the difference. But you do and the value your practice brings to the table is what separates you from the rest.

The options are endless so find your niche, passion, and purpose. Take full ownership of being the best in your market for your niche. A bit of time invested in researching your market area will provide the understanding necessary to dominate. There are a wealth of tools and technologies that can show you the exact demographic that is consuming the types of dental service you want to hone in on. If you don't know who your avatar is, your efforts to capture them as patients will come up short.

Do This

- • Clearly define your niche
- • Research and understand who your ideal patient is (avatar)
- • Own this area of dental expertise and enjoy being the go-to practice for your niche

Photo Credit: Bigstock

Beyond Minimalism

Beyond Minimalism

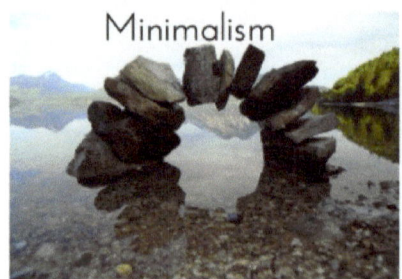

Dental Practice Resource Group

Minimalism can simplify your life, but it's not what the patient is hoping for.

If you want your practice to stand out and rise to the top, you must deliver well beyond the minimal requirements. Satisfied and average are indicative of mediocrity. Taking things up even a small notch creates a lasting impression in your patient's mind. Build on that each and every time, and you will create self-perpetuating loyalty.

In today's age, social media reigns supreme. My 85 year old father-in-law is a Facebook junkie, and chances are most of your patients have their favorite social media app as well. This is a perfect opportunity for free marketing.

Over time, patients become like friends and family. For example, Leesa has been coming to our practice for years. She is a bit of a self-proclaimed worrier and appreciates a warm neck wrap with a few drops of lemon oil. The calming effect is noticed by all. Our team reviews the current day's patients and makes sure that her scented neck wrap is ready as soon as she hits the chair. We've seen her positive comments and even a few selfies posted on Facebook and Instagram from her visits. This simple act takes only a few minutes but has created a raving fan who has referred dozens of friends to our practice.

Do This:

- Be so good they can't ignore you
- Don't accept satisfied and average as end points
- Plan the day to reward patients with small gestures
- Aim for the next level of patient experience and personalize your care

Photo credit: BigStock

Step Out Of The Way

Step Out Of The Way

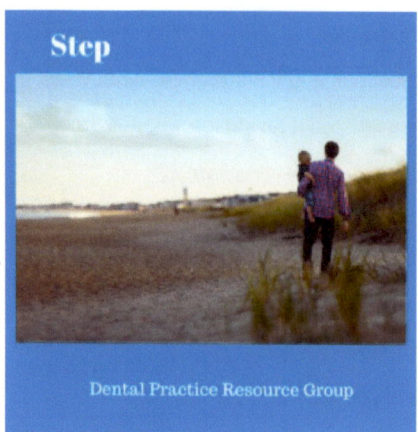

Creating a workflow that simplifies how you do business as an important element that is often approached from the wrong direction. While having processes and procedures that allow efficiency and ease for your team, realize that the same may not hold true for the patients.

Ask these question:

If I were the patient, would it be easy to engage and do business with this dental practice?

Do they make it easy for me to complete my forms?

What about insurance forms and assistance with other paperwork?

Are they friendly when I call with a question or concern?

Let Them Lead

We simply ask our patients how they prefer to complete required forms. The results from last years' data shows that 64% prefer to complete their health history, contact information and update insurance policy information online. Our team added this option to the patient portal with a bit of help from our webmaster. The paper forms are still available for the rest who prefer to share their data that way.

We found that allowing online access to update insurance information saves the front desk staff countless hours on the phone and helps us get paid.

Do This:

- Think of how a patient would feel when crafting policy and procedures
- Understand that the digital age can streamline your workflow and patients love the option
- Ask: Is this making it easier for the patient to engage and interact with the practice?
-

Photo credit: s-danielle-macinnes

Inside Knowledge

Inside Information

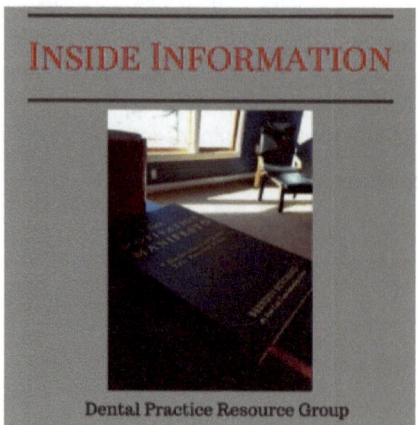

Have you ever had molar endo or a Gow-Gates block? If so, you have the power of insight and can share first-hand experience with patients.

When your team knows first-hand how a procedure is supposed to go or what an appliance feels like, patients respond with trust and feel reassured when facing an upcoming procedure.

Know The Next Step

I called our Vet recently after a minor eye issue turned ugly. The doctor was out that afternoon, but his office manager returned my call and shared what typically happens next. She prefaced her comments with that fact she'd be running it by the doctor tomorrow but wanted to give me an idea that surgery would be needed. When the Vet called back the next day, I wasn't in shock about having to drive 200 miles to see an animal eye specialist and that surgery was performed that same afternoon.

Patients often have questions long after the dentist has stepped out of the room. They call back nervous, worried or in a panic wanting information. By teaching your staff the next step in the process, you have created a system to keep patients happy and loyal.

Common examples in our practice include:

-When will the oral surgeon place the implant?

-How soon can I get a tooth on my implant?

-What does Invisalign feel like when changing trays?

-I've been referred to the endodontist, what can I expect?

Our practice has a lot of Invisalign cases, and one of our hygienists made a few videos sharing what to expect, caring for the trays and a time-lapse video showing her progress.

Do This:
- Teach your staff the next step or two in the process
- Share honest experiences when possible and help patients understand what to expect
- Making any experience as smooth as possible for the patient will further grow your positive reputation as a practice that delivers amazing care

Serving Happiness

Serving Happiness

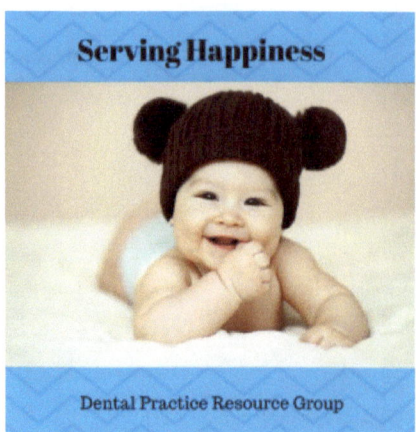

Doesn't it feel good when a patient expresses their gratitude and appreciation for the care you provide? Human nature craves wanting and appreciation. Take this opportunity to pay it backward. Let your patients know that you appreciate them as well.

We have covered many ideas and methods to develop loyalty, and many of these same techniques let patients know you appreciate them.

Here is what our practice does routinely to express gratitude:

-Verbally thank the patient

-Send thank you cards to all new patients for choosing our practice

-Handwritten notes for special events in our patients' lives

-Free whitening for brides

-Open office policy and patients routinely stop by for a Keurig coffee

-Patient appreciation days with treats from a local bakery or deli

Do This:

- Reward your patients for being patients
- Show appreciation in a way that fits with your local customs
- Communicate thanks through notes, phone calls and social media presence

Photo credit: Bigstock

Gather The Unsatisfied And

Gather The Unsatisfied And...

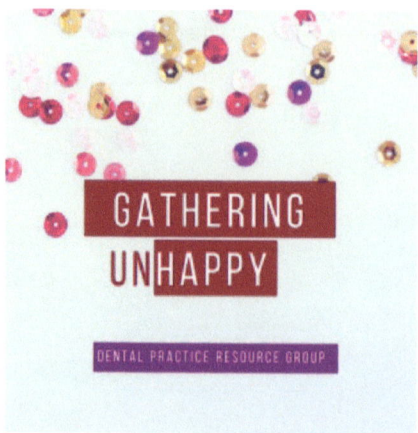

The market allows patients to pick and choose where they receive care for the most part. When patients are unhappy, they leave and come to your door. Take this chance and deliver excellence from the first contact with your practice.

This book has stressed the creation of an experience vastly different from the average dental practice. When the entire team focuses on designing an amazing experience instead of just an extraction or crown prep, patients sit up and take notice.

Find Their Need

Patients leave practices for a variety of reasons but not having their needs met is at the top. When new patients show up, we always ask how or why they came to our practice. Knowing this information up front lets us tailor their experience to ensure we are not only meeting, but exceeding those needs. It is a simple question and one they often appreciate being asked. It also lets us know other areas of opportunity based on where other local practices have let patients down.

Make It Easy

Our team does whatever it takes to make a new patient feel welcome and smooth their transition into our practice. We help them transfer records, ask about their specific needs and work to deliver an amazing experience. Our team is deliberate about making them feel at home and appreciated from day one.

Do This:

- Deliver an amazing experience in areas your competitors fails
- Understand that chance is not a friend - create a script and process that impresses new patients

Average Law

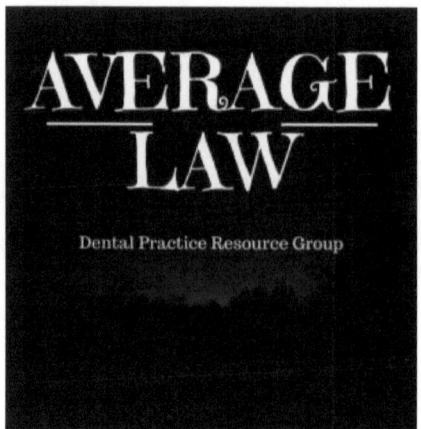

Throughout this book, we have emphasized creating an amazing experience but also realize we all are only human. Mistakes happen, interactions don't go as planned and patients become upset. This is the price of doing business in healthcare.

While the goal is always to be on the mark, consistency is the equalizer. When patients are consistently impressed by the practice, they overlook or forget moments that disappointed.

Be on the lookout for any opportunity to shine. A few minutes of doing what the patient did not expect erases doubt and elevates your status in the patients' minds.

Here is a recent example from our practice:

John is a sporadic patient in our practice and no longer drives due to a stroke. He used public transportation to make his appointments and was referred to an oral surgeon for a difficult extraction. He called for his ride, but it became apparent that he was going to miss his appointment. One of our team members drove him to the oral surgeon's office and waited until he was seen. She then called his transportation service and explained the situation. They sent a driver over quickly, and he was able to leave as soon as his oral surgery procedure was over.

Do This:

- Be consistent and step up whenever the opportunity to be amazing presents itself
- Surprise patients and do things they don't expect
- Know that the law of averages applies and make up for shortcomings by focusing on the unique needs of individual patients

Checking In

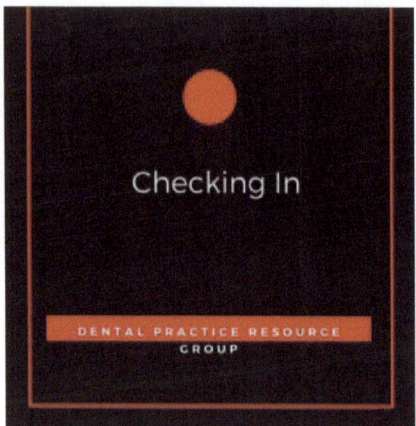

Following up with patients establishes confidence in your caring. This simple strategy is often overlooked or labeled a waste of time.

Don't make it a burden. These calls are short and to the point. Expressing concern is a welcome sentiment and lets the patient know your practice cares and is grateful.

Other times a note will suffice and on specific occasions, a social media comment goes a long way to letting the patient know you are interested in them for more than collecting a fee.

Several of our staff are savvy social media users and keep up with local high school and college sports teams. They chime in and share congrats or words of encouragement on Facebook and other platforms. Many of our patients play on those teams, and it is an easy way to stay engaged with the community and our patients.

Do This:

- Check-in and follow-up with patients
- Send notes congratulating patients for events such as honor roll, graduation, sporting wins
- Harness the power of social media and be where your patients can see you

Unfinal Touch

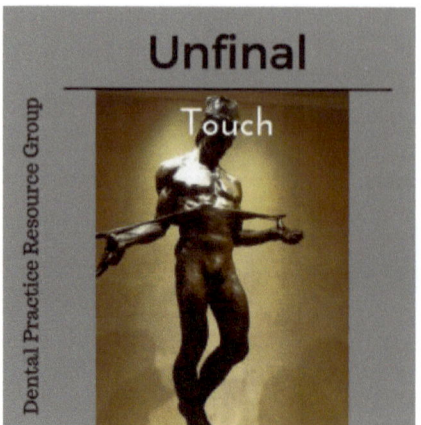

In the last section, we talked about what to do after the fact. This chapter focuses on keeping top of mind.

We are realists and know that going to the dentist, or thinking about the dental office for that matter, is far from a top priority for most patients. We carefully plan and encourage six-month hygiene checks, but once patients walk out that door the information seems to evaporate.

Our practice uses a variety of tools and techniques to gently remind patients we are here for them.

We have a bi-weekly column in the local newspaper called "Ask The Expert." In a short 250-word article, we share a variety of tips on keeping a healthy smile. The team member who writes the article has their picture and our logo included.

We have monthly Facebook contests and encourage patients to "Like Us." We give out movie passes, gift cards, restaurant passes, and occasionally iPods and electric toothbrushes.

Our monthly e-newsletter shares tips on remaining healthy and aging gracefully. We share tips from physicians, age researchers, nutritionists and physical therapists.

Our team volunteers at local events such as Give Kids A Smile, community homeless shelter events, and charity events. We even created a running team and participated in local 5 and 10K events. We have won the largest team award four times in as many years. Our brightly colored shirts are proudly worn by patients and have been posted on Facebook from sites around the world, courtesy of a high school patient on a European Tour.

Do This:
- Look for opportunities for the practice to be seen
- Be part of the local color and show up to help others
- Educate, support and entertain the local community
- Share your team and talents
-

Ready?

Ready To Begin?

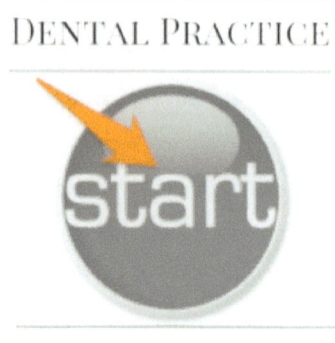

You are part of something amazing and have the opportunity to change lives every day. Not many professions can say that. Your patients like and trust that you will competently solve their oral health issues, but when you go beyond the expected your reputation will soar.

While not every example shared in this book applies to your practice, use the creativity of your team to design an experience that values and rewards the patient. Show them you actually care and are invested in them beyond collecting a fee.

Dentistry often gets a bad rap. Use this as a chance to change the perception by delivering an amazing experience every patient, every time. Step into the public spotlight and let the local community you care about them, whether they are your patient or not.

Now that you're done reading this, take a few moments and pick one or two strategies that spoke to you. Bring your ideas back to your team and begin to create your unique brand of delivering dental care. Be confident in using the tools you have learned and distinguish your practice as the best place to be a dental patient.